WELCOME

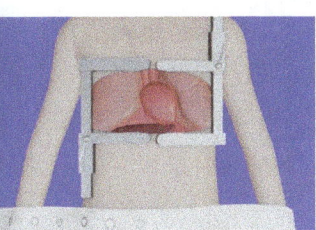

1st Edition 2021

Authors: Nick Chilvers, Ben Wooldridge, Matthew Wyse and Joel Dunning.

Produced by Nick Chilvers

Forward

Welcome to the Resuscitative Thoracotomy – A Team Approach course. This handbook is designed to supplement the pre-course e-learning and the interactive course itself. These protocols have been compiled following many years of learning from experience and collaborative discussions with emergency and pre-hospital physicians, nurses, paramedics and allied health professionals, anaesthetists, intensivists and surgeons. We aim to provide you with a detailed overview of the current evidence in this field and to discuss the technical aspects of resuscitative thoracotomies and the clinical management of these patients. Furthermore, we will cover some of the more difficult, special circumstances and focus on the teamwork and human factors that play such a key role in these challenging scenarios. The latter will be consolidated by moulages during the second half of the course. Please note the purpose of the course is not so much a focus on the procedure of resuscitative thoracotomy itself, nor does it certify you as competent in performing one. There are multiple courses, mainly cadaveric, that already offer these opportunities. Rather, we aim to explore the human factors and wider skills required to manage these patients, as well as providing structure to the resuscitation as a whole, which we feel is unique to this course. Furthermore, this course is designed to provide skills and protocols that can be used in conjunction with those already learnt from ATLS or the European Trauma Course that you employ every day.

We hope that you enjoy the course and that the knowledge and skills you gain improve your confidence in looking after these complex patients. However, we strongly recommend that you incorporate such training into your own units, as we believe that it is only by practising moulages that we can ensure that the wider team feels confident and are thus able to give patients the best possible outcome when they come through the door.

About us

We are a group of clinicians including emergency physicians, pre-hospital physicians, anaesthetists, cardiothoracic surgeons and specialist allied health professionals who are passionate about improving the care and outcomes of trauma patients. Courses will always be delivered by a mixed team, including cardiothoracic surgeons, providing delegates with the best learning opportunity.

Recommended Resources

A list of references can be found at the end of this document and any key resources are highlighted in the text.

Top tips
Special 'top tips' boxes like this can be found throughout the text to highlight key points or provide extra information

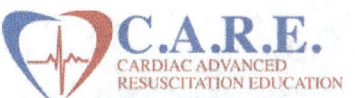

Please join us on Facebook for further information

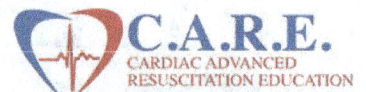

CONTENTS

Resuscitative Thoracotomy: The Evidence	1
Lessons from Real Life: An Emergency Thoracotomy	7
Technical Aspects of a Resuscitative Thoracotomy	8
Resuscitative Thoracotomy Equipment	11
Working as a Team in Resuscitative Thoracotomy: The Protocol	13
Performing the Resuscitative Thoracotomy	21
The Timeout and Beyond in Resuscitative Thoracotomy	28
Non-arrest Situations in Penetrating Thoracic Trauma	30
Special Circumstances in Thoracic Trauma	34
Moulages: Putting it all into Practice	40
Human Factors in Resuscitative Thoracotomy	41
References	45
Notes	47

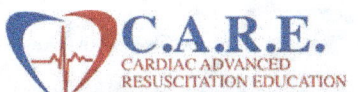

RESUSCITATIVE THORACOTOMY: THE EVIDENCE

eLearning Module 1

The evidence surrounding resuscitative thoracotomy is reasonably limited. Although there are a few areas where there seems to be reasonable consensus, for example its efficacy in a recent arrest from penetrating chest trauma, there is a lot of debate and variation between centres. Indeed, there is no strict protocol in Europe or internationally. Herein, we describe the best current evidence and discuss some of the areas of contention.

The first place to refer to regarding governance of resuscitation in Europe is the European Resuscitation Council (ERC) Guidelines for Resuscitation 2021[1] (an update on the original 2015 Guidelines)[2], which are supported by Resus Council UK. The recent update followed multiple systematic reviews of the literature. There have been a few changes, but the majority of the guidelines reinforce/substantiate the 2015 guidelines. The 'Special Circumstances' section includes a flow chart for traumatic arrest including resuscitative thoracotomy (see below).

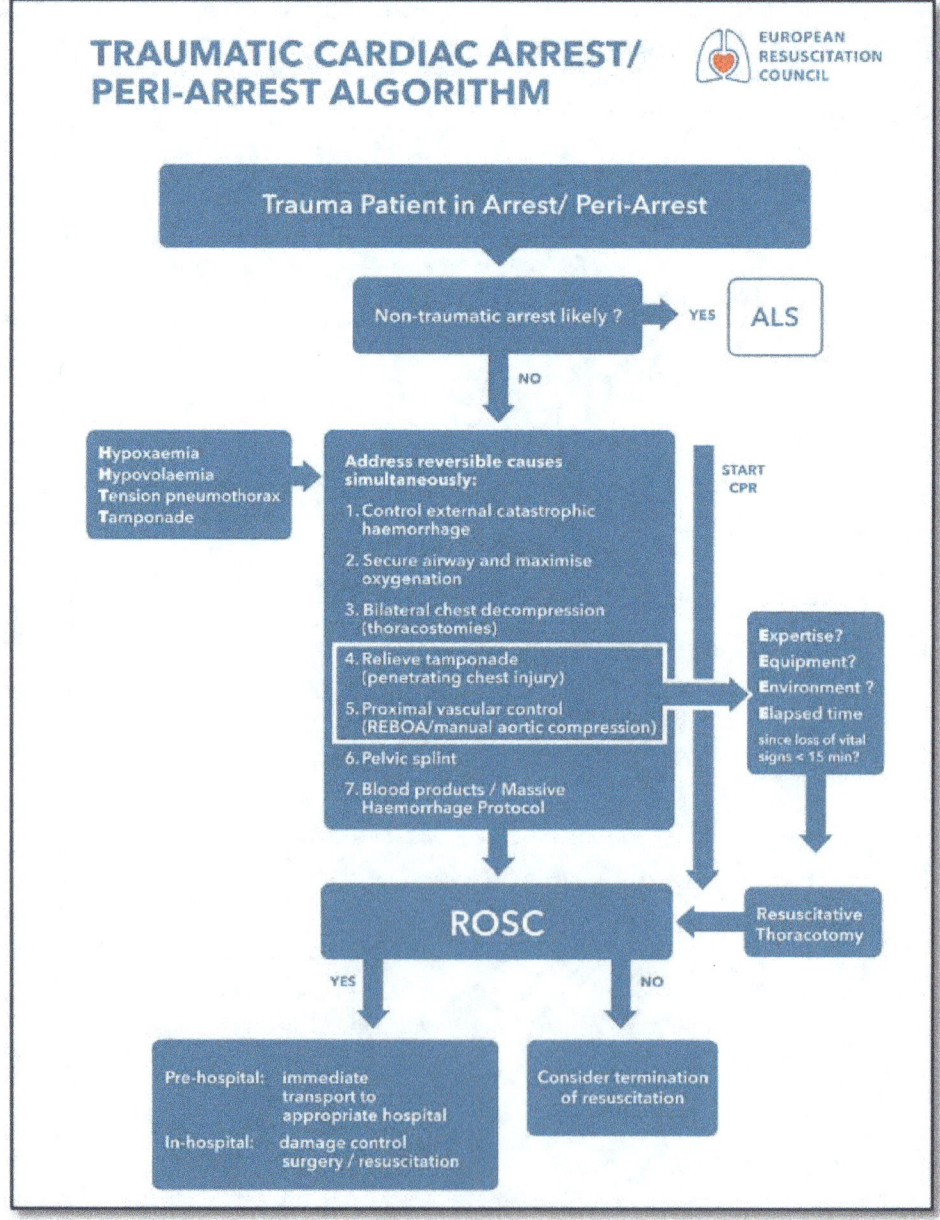

European Resuscitation Council Traumatic Cardiac Arrest Algorithm 2021[1]

The guidelines ask you to initially consider the likelihood of arrest being secondary to trauma. If so, then this is where there is a deviation from the standard ALS protocols. In particular, consider diagnoses of tension pneumothorax, tamponade, hypoxia and hypovolaemia and consider the need for a resuscitative thoracotomy. The ERC guidelines also make recommendations about which patients would benefit. In summary they suggest that resuscitative thoracotomy is indicated if it is:

- within **15 minutes** of loss of vital signs **whether penetrating or blunt trauma**[1]

However, they do note that the outcomes following resuscitative thoracotomy are particularly poor for blunt trauma. Regarding penetrating trauma, they found that stabbing has better prognosis than other mechanisms.

They also give guidance to say that unless their 'four E's rule' is met then resuscitative thoracotomy should not be attempted.[1,2] These are:

- **Expertise**
- **Equipment**
- **Environment**: Ideally operating theatre or location equipped to perform thoracotomy
- **Elapsed Time**: Thoracotomy should be performed within the stated timeframes

The four Es is really what this course is all about and why it has been established. Although we have less influence on the elapsed time (other than through educating prehospital care teams and the public to transport these patients as quickly as possible and ensure that there is quick decision making in the emergency department), with relevant training and equipment the first three can be addressed.

A particular emphasis is placed on the simultaneous treatment of reversible causes being the first priority and use of ultrasound is recommended to aid diagnosis and guide emergency management. This is where it is key to appreciate the difference in aetiologies of traumatic compared to medical cardiac arrest. For the former, the most common reversible causes are uncontrolled haemorrhage (48%), tension pneumothorax (13%), asphyxia (13%) and pericardial tamponade (10%), with arrest rhythms of PEA and asystole in the majority (66% and 30% respectively).[1] Hence, treatment of reversible causes e.g. establishing an airway, controlling external haemorrhage, chest decompression and possible resuscitative thoracotomy, take priority over chest compressions. Furthermore, chest compressions will not be as effective as in normovolaemia/non-traumatic arrests; "don't pump an empty heart"[1] and open cardiac massage following resuscitative thoracotomy provides a more favourable outcome. The ERC 2021 guidelines recommend withholding resuscitation if there are "no signs of life within the preceding 15 mins [or] massive trauma incompatible with survival" and termination if, once all reversible causes are addressed, there is no ROSC or no cardiac activity on ultrasound.

Regarding chest decompression in traumatic arrest, the guidelines suggest bilateral 4th intercostal space thoracostomies. These are more likely to be effective than needle decompression during positive pressure ventilation, can be extended into a clamshell and are quicker than tube thoracostomies. When ventilating, it is advised to monitor and aim for normocapnia and to consider low tidal volumes, as this may improve cardiac preload.

A final important recommendation is for "immediate aortic occlusion… as a last resort measure in patients with exsanguinating and uncontrollable infra-diaphragmatic torso haemorrhage" either by directly cross clamping following a resuscitative thoracotomy or with the use of Resuscitative Endovascular Balloon Occlusion of the Aorta (REBOA). Their review of the literature found no evidence of either being superior.[1,3]

The Royal College of Emergency Medicine (UK) published a best practice guideline for Cardiac Arrest in Adults in 2019.[4] Much of the content and their algorithm (right) are similar to the ERC guidelines. In particular, they too emphasise the importance in traumatic arrests of prioritising initial lifesaving interventions to treat reversible causes over external chest compressions, vasopressors and defibrillation. The algorithm also calls for early ultrasound, which can assist in diagnosing tamponade, detecting cardiac activity and assessing cardiac filling. Finally, they recommend departments have their own clear protocols for resuscitative thoracotomy incorporating the available resources and staff skillsets within that centre. We believe this point is particularly crucial. Indeed, one of the purposes of this course is to encourage your department to develop their own local guidelines informed by the knowledge and skills that this course has to offer.

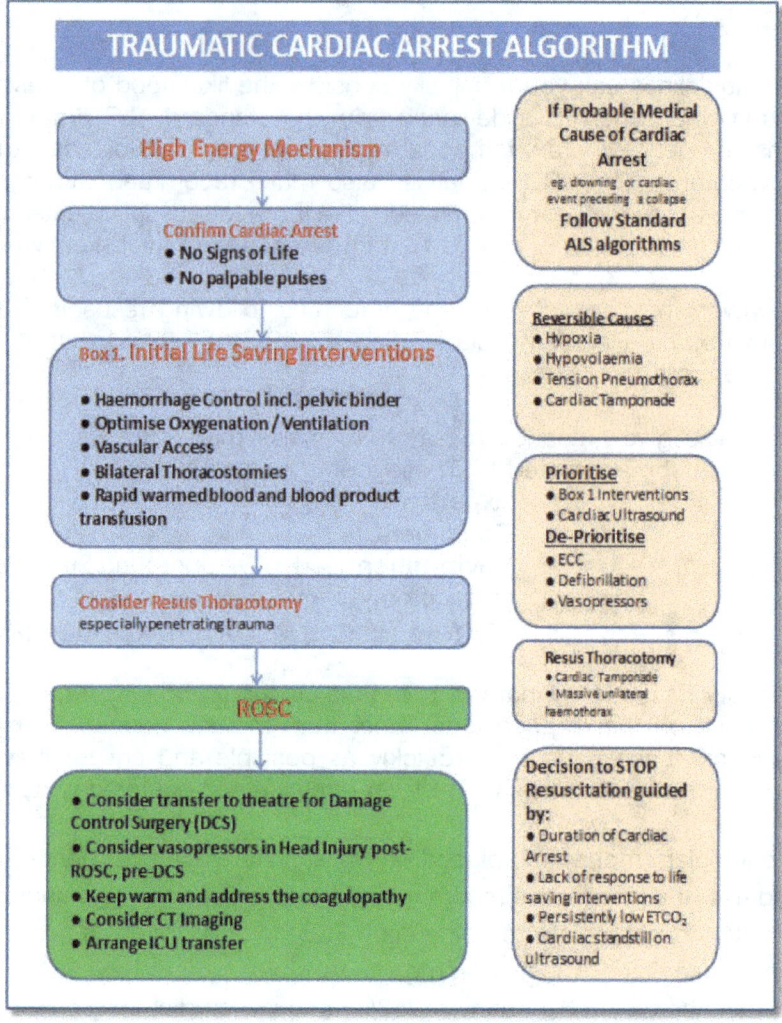

Traumatic cardiac arrest algorithm RCEM 2019[4]

Elsewhere, the American Heart Association published some brief guidelines in 2010,[5] reissued in 2015,[6] and also state that resuscitative thoracotomy may be indicated in selected patients. They refer to the American College of Surgeons committee on trauma, which found a survival of 7.8% (11.2% penetrating, 1.6% blunt trauma),[5] which concurs with the European guidelines[1] in that blunt trauma has a poor outcome. One should note that, compared to the UK, the US has a higher proportion of gunshots compared to stabbings and this may be why their survival for penetrating trauma is lower. The guidelines also refer to the criteria for terminating resuscitation by the Emergency Medical Services (EMS) physicians[7] which are discussed in due course. Finally, for tamponade they recommend that emergency department thoracotomy may improve survival in patients who are in arrest, or peri-arrest, compared to pericardiocentesis due to the likelihood of clotted blood in the pericardial sac.

The American College of Surgeons (ACS) Practice management guidelines for Emergency Department Thoracotomy 2001[8] is probably the most extensive international guidelines for Emergency Department Thoracotomy. The guidelines include a full literature review with evidence-based recommendations. Unsurprisingly, there is no level I evidence given the nature of this topic, which does not lend itself well to randomised controlled trials.

The ACS guidelines[8] do however find sufficient level II evidence to make the following recommendations:

Level II

1. Emergency department thoracotomy should be performed rarely in patients sustaining cardiopulmonary arrest secondary to blunt trauma because of its very low survival rate and poor neurologic outcomes. It should be limited to those that arrive with vital signs at the trauma center and experience a *witnessed* cardiopulmonary arrest.
2. Emergency department thoracotomy is best applied to patients sustaining penetrating cardiac injuries who arrive at trauma centers after a short scene and transport time with witnessed or objectively measured physiologic parameters (signs of life): pupillary response, spontaneous ventilation, presence of carotid pulse, measurable or palpable blood pressure, extremity movement, and cardiac electrical activity.
3. Emergency department thoracotomy should be performed in patients sustaining penetrating noncardiac thoracic injuries, but these patients generally experience a low survival rate. Because it is difficult to ascertain whether the injuries are noncardiac thoracic versus cardiac, emergency department thoracotomy can be used to establish the diagnosis.
4. Emergency department thoracotomy should be performed in patients sustaining exsanguinating abdominal vascular injuries, but these patients generally experience a low survival rate. Judicious selection of patients should be exercised. This procedure should be used as an adjunct to definitive repair of the abdominal-vascular injury.
5. For the pediatric population guidelines 1-4 are applicable.

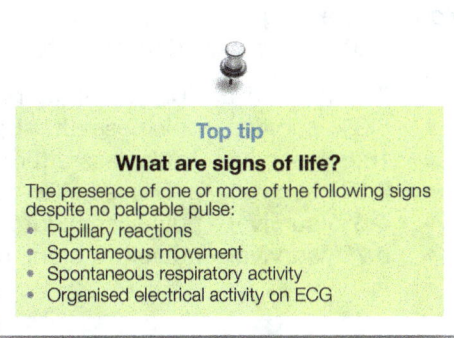

Top tip
What are signs of life?
The presence of one or more of the following signs despite no palpable pulse:
- Pupillary reactions
- Spontaneous movement
- Spontaneous respiratory activity
- Organised electrical activity on ECG

Recommendations from *The American College of Surgeons Practice management guidelines for Emergency Department Thoracotomy 2001*[8]

In summary, they also agree that resuscitative thoracotomy is most successful in cases of penetrating trauma and only rarely in blunt trauma. They support its use in non-cardiac penetrating thoracic injuries but advise caution in exsanguinating abdominal injuries and appreciate the poor outcomes in these patients. In this latter group the problem is not in the chest and cross clamping the aorta may buy time, but there needs to be a definitive intervention to an amenable injury. The other of their points to note is that short downtimes with evidence of signs of life (see above) will give the best outcomes and this should be borne in mind when formulating individual unit guidelines. We would also support their final recommendation regarding paediatrics.[8] These patients have the same mechanisms of injury and the same (maybe even better) chance of survival.

The AHA publication referred to the 2003 National Association of EMS Physicians (NAEMSP) Standards and Clinical Practice Committee and the ACS Committee on Trauma – Guidelines for withholding or termination of resuscitation in prehospital cardiopulmonary arrest.[7] The association performed a literature review that included 2691 patients. 1746 suffered penetrating trauma, of which 16% (276) survived, whilst the remainder suffered blunt trauma with a survival of only 2%.[7]

They conclude that patients who have had penetrating trauma, but who are found to be pulseless and apnoeic but have signs of life should be resuscitated. Situations where resuscitation shouldn't be considered or should be withdrawn include:
- Blunt trauma victims with no signs of life
- Witnessed arrest and more than 15 minutes of unsuccessful CPR or more than a 15 minute transfer time to the ED
- Victims with injuries incompatible with life such as decapitation or hemicorporectomy

The second point is particularly important, as if the patient has exsanguinated or tamponaded then external cardiac massage is not effective and vital organs will be starved of oxygen. This once again highlights the importance of only considering patients for resuscitative thoracotomy who have recently suffered arrest.

The Eastern Association for the Surgery of Trauma has produced a practice management guideline for patient selection for emergency department thoracotomy (EDT).[9] The great strength of their literature review is the large number of patients (10,238 from 72 studies) and subdivision based on clinical presentation. This review demonstrated the following findings:

- 21.3% survival – pulseless after penetrating injury (signs of life)
- 8.3% survival – pulseless after penetrating injury (no signs of life)
- 15.6% survival – pulseless after penetrating extra-thoracic injury (signs of life)
- 2.9% survival – pulseless after penetrating extra-thoracic injury (no signs of life)
- 4.6% survival – pulseless blunt injury (signs of life)
- 0.7% survival – pulseless blunt injury (no signs of life)

Question	Recommendation
PICO #1	In patients who present pulseless to the Emergency Department with signs of life after penetrating thoracic injury, we **strongly recommend** resuscitative Emergency Department thoracotomy. **Strong Recommendation**
PICO #2	In patients who present pulseless to the Emergency Department without signs of life after penetrating thoracic injury, we **conditionally recommend** resuscitative Emergency Department thoracotomy. **Conditional Recommendation**
PICO #3	In patients who present pulseless to the Emergency Department with signs of life after penetrating extra-thoracic injury, we **conditionally recommend** resuscitative Emergency Department thoracotomy. **Conditional Recommendation**
PICO #4	In patients who present pulseless to the Emergency Department without signs of life after penetrating extra-thoracic injury, we **conditionally recommend** resuscitative Emergency Department thoracotomy.[1] **Conditional Recommendation**
PICO #5	In patients who present pulseless to the Emergency Department with signs of life after blunt injury, we **conditionally recommend** resuscitative Emergency Department thoracotomy. **Conditional Recommendation**
PICO #6	In patients who present pulseless to the Emergency Department without signs of life after blunt injury, we **conditionally recommend against** resuscitative Emergency Department thoracotomy.[2] **Conditional Recommendation**

Figure 7. Final recommendations. [1]Group voting for a recommendation was mixed. While all voted for a "conditional" recommendation, 11 members voted in favor of Emergency Department Thoracotomy and 4 voted against the procedure based on the PICO #4 Evidence Profile. [2]Group voting for a recommendation was mixed. While all voted against the performance of Emergency Department Thoracotomy based on the PICO #6 Evidence Profile, 10 members voted for a "strong" recommendation and 5 voted for a "conditional" recommendation.

Recommendations from *An evidence-based approach to patient selection for emergency department thoracotomy: A practice management guideline from the Eastern Association for the Surgery of Trauma 2015.*[9]

This large study once again concurs that the best outcomes are in patients with penetrating trauma who present with signs of life and strongly recommended EDT, whilst they conditionally recommended it for patients without signs of life. Penetrating extra-thoracic injury was found to be a heterogenous group and they conditionally recommended EDT with signs of life but recognised different injury patterns may not have equivalent salvage rates. The evidence was low quality for patients without signs of life and there was disagreement within their group leading to a conditional recommendation for EDT. The guideline recognises the poor outcomes in blunt trauma but conditionally recommend EDT if signs of life. However, they appreciated that many patients would not wish for this due to poor neurological outcomes, which are worse than in penetrating trauma victims. Finally, for blunt trauma without signs of life they conditionally recommend against EDT. Indeed only 1 patient out of 825 pulseless blunt trauma patients presenting with no signs of life survived without neurological impairment.[9]

Summary of evidence discussed so far

The overriding message from all of these guidelines is that resuscitative thoracotomy should be performed in patients suffering from penetrating trauma with recent arrest. There is potentially a role for resuscitative thoracotomy in extra-thoracic penetrating trauma and in blunt trauma victims with signs of life, however, the evidence suggests that we should be selective. Several groups suggest that resuscitative thoracotomy should not be performed in blunt trauma with no signs of life.

What is lacking in these guidelines is direction for events following the decision to do a resuscitative thoracotomy and indeed this is where the literature is fairly thin. There are some reasonable recommendations about which patients it is indicated for and how likely it is to work but not so much on what to do next. Before we proceed with our protocol, we will quickly consider the few papers that are published to see what other groups recommend.

Protocols for resuscitative thoracotomy

The Royal Melbourne Hospital published a comprehensive Emergency Department Thoracotomy Guideline in 2011.[10] These state clear indications for resuscitative thoracotomy in the arrested patient with tamponade but also for peri-arrest patients with refractory shock despite chest decompression and trauma resuscitation, with evidence of cardiac activity and tamponade on echocardiogram. Of note, their contraindications include lack of training. However, the strength of this publication is a detailed step by step description of how to perform the resuscitative thoracotomy and an equipment list.

In the UK, the South Yorkshire Major Trauma Operational Delivery Network has created a network guideline for resuscitative thoracotomy.[11] Similar to the Melbourne publication,[10] they have outlined who will benefit, provide an equipment list and describe how to perform the procedure. They recommend a clamshell for all patients and, for a number of reasons, this is what we are recommending in our protocol. These guidelines were based on a fantastic paper published in the Emergency Medicine Journal entitled "Emergency thoracotomy: "how to do it"".[12]

Pre-Hospital resuscitative thoracotomy

Most physician staffed air ambulance teams have a pre-hospital thoracotomy Standard Operating Procedure (SOP). The Faculty of Pre-Hospital Care (Royal College of Surgeons Ed) have produced consensus guidelines,[13] that unsurprisingly reflect much of the evidence discussed above, and support the practice of performing resuscitative thoracotomy via a clamshell incision at the earliest opportunity. This practice means that in communities served by physician staffed pre-hospital teams it is important to prepare for patients who may arrive in the Emergency Department with the chest already open.

Summary

The evidence has shown that in blunt trauma the chance of success is slim, with survival of 0.7-4.6%.[9] There is therefore a need to be highly selective, especially if the patient has already arrested rather than arresting in front of you. Extra-thoracic trauma patients also have inferior outcomes and we would also advise careful thought before undertaking the procedure in this situation. As discussed previously, the ERC guidelines do support aortic occlusion, either via thoracotomy or REBOA, as a last resort for infra-diaphragmatic trauma.[1] The best outcomes are in penetrating thoracic trauma, particularly if the injury is to the heart, with recent arrest or refractory shock. Although all the evidence discussed above is of great value in helping us to make informed decisions and has provided detail on how to perform a resuscitative thoracotomy, there is a need for a protocol to describe the overall process of managing these patients. This course aims to instruct you in organising your team and managing the patient from receiving them through the door to transferring them to theatre.

LEARNING FROM REAL LIFE: AN EMERGENCY THORACOTOMY

eLearning Module 2

Given the low volume of major chest traumas in most UK centres, learning from the experience of others is particularly important. *eLearning module 2* explains how you can access a video of a real-life thoracotomy from St Vincent's Hospital, Sydney.

This is probably the best available example of a real-life thoracotomy. The patient had sustained penetrating trauma and presented with signs of life but was tamponading and subsequently arrested in ED. Following a left thoracotomy, the surgeon decompressed the tamponade and placed a thumb over a hole in the left ventricle. The incision was then extended to a clamshell and a foley catheter placed through the hole and inflated. This provided some control of the bleeding and allowed the surgeon to then suture the hole.

The video demonstrates strong leadership and communication, both within the ED team and with other teams, including the theatre team. There are some profound points to note from this video. Preparation is extremely important, as is having the right equipment and knowing what is in your trays. The team did very well but were hampered slightly by the equipment available and the time taken to acquire this. They improvised well, but it is clear that a dedicated resuscitative thoracotomy tray containing everything the surgeon needed would have been of great help. Finally, the surgeon was assisted by a colleague who had never seen or practiced resuscitative thoracotomy.

By practising in simulations multiple times, we can be prepared for patients who come in more emergently e.g. with prehospital cardiac arrest and lacking the preparation time that they had in this scenario. By ensuring the ED has the correct trays and that the wider team knows what equipment is available and has practised how the procedure is performed, we can improve the confidence of everyone involved.

TECHNICAL ASPECTS OF A RESUSCITATIVE THORACOTOMY
eLearning Modules 3a/3b/4

eLearning Modules 3a and 3b comprise 8 videos that clearly demonstrate the steps in resuscitative thoracotomy and important related skills. We have summarised the key learning points below.

Video 1 - Left anterior thoracotomy

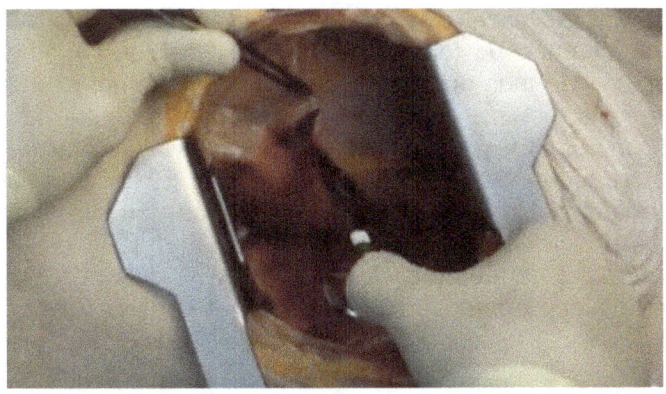

An incision is made in the pericardium medial to the phrenic nerve

Note that we recommend a full clamshell but, nonetheless, this video displays the anatomy clearly. You can clearly see the surgeon going through each layer quickly but in a controlled fashion. The phrenic nerve is seen on the pericardium and an incision made medially to relieve any tamponade. Exposure is key; make the thoracotomy as large as you can – all the way to the sternum and posteriorly as far as you can. A trained assistant can perform the same on the right and the two joined by dividing the sternum, with a Gigli saw or plaster shears, to complete the clamshell.

Video 2 - Internal cardiac massage

This video demonstrates internal cardiac massage. The right hand is placed behind the heart, as far up as you can. Put the left hand flat on the front of the heart and squeeze, 'milking' the blood from the apex upwards at around 80-100 beats per minute. Never dip your thumb or finger tips into the heart as it can tear through. Be mindful to keep the heart as horizontal as possible and not lift it vertically, as this can obstruct flow.

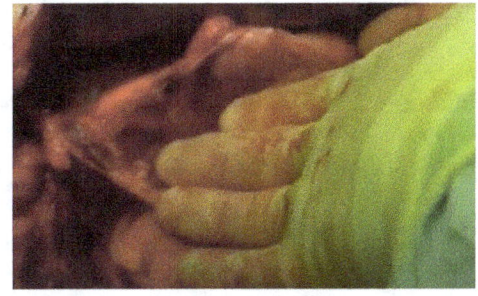

A flat hand is used to internally massage the heart

Video 3 - Clamping the descending aorta

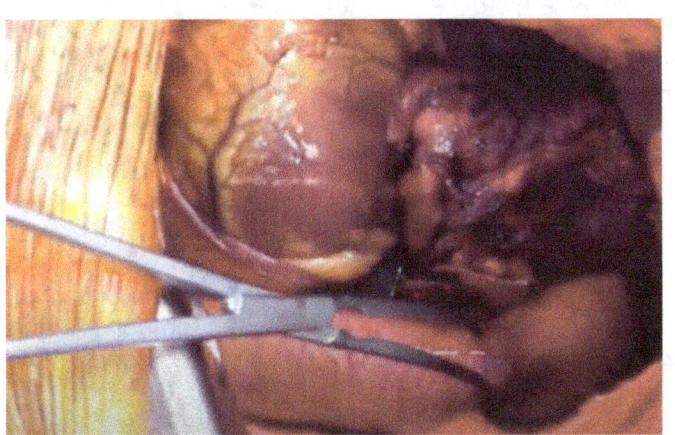

A clamp is applied to the descending aorta

This video demonstrates how a clamp can be applied to the descending aorta through the left side of the chest. It is not necessary to get all the way around the back of the vessel as there are other branches coming off. There is also a risk of damaging other structures such as the oesophagus if placed too far into the mediastinum. A clamp positioned most of the way across the aorta or a fist compressing it against the spine should improve the blood pressure to the upper body.

Video 4 – Sternotomy for midline stab injury

This video demonstrates how a more stable patient might be treated after being transferred to theatre. The tamponade is initially relieved by opening the pericardium from a subxiphoid incision. The incision is subsequently extended into a median sternotomy, which cardiac surgeons use for the majority of their operations. In theatre there is specialist equipment not available in the emergency department, specifically diathermy, a sternal saw, cell salvage and cardiopulmonary bypass facilities.

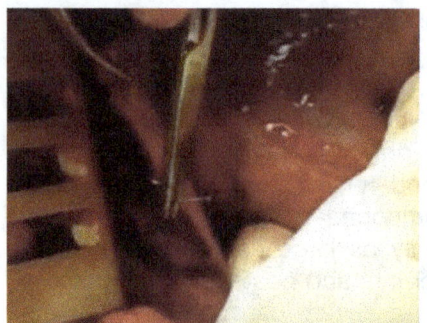

A myocardial injury is sutured

There are some key technical elements that are highlighted in the video. The retractor must be fully closed before insertion into the chest. The operator can then open the retractor, although not all the way at this stage. As the tissues adjust and settle the retractor can gradually be opened further. If your view is poor, always consider increasing the retraction or extending the incision. The heart is covered by pericardium, fatty tissue and, in this case, mediastinal haematoma. The pericardium is opened in the midline to avoid the phrenic nerves. Finally, sutures are placed to close a defect in the beating heart. The video demonstrates how difficult this is, even for heart surgeons.

Video 5 – Urgent left thoracotomy in a patient with an output

This video demonstrates a fast left thoracotomy using a scalpel. The operator makes an incision curving up into the axilla in the direction of the ribs and uses the scalpel all the way down to the ribs and intercostal spaces. Scissors, with a finger behind to prevent damage to the lung, are used to divide the intercostal muscles. A retractor provides access to the chest, but you can appreciate that exposure is limited. This patient is relatively stable with an output and so the chest is then packed in preparation for cardiothoracic surgeons to provide definitive surgical management of the injuries.

Video 6 – Left thoracotomy and opening of pericardium

The operator in this video doesn't have a finger behind his scissors so could be at risk of damaging the lung. The retractor is also placed upside down and will limit his access, particularly if extension to a clamshell is required. What is performed well however, is access into the pericardium. The operator lifts up the pericardium with two instruments and then safely cuts through the tented part. We would then recommend opening the pericardium fully, allowing two handed pericardial massage.

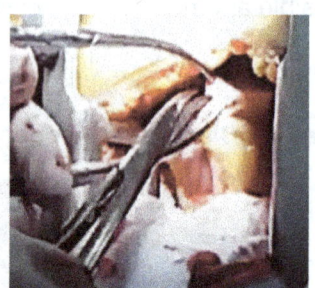

The pericardium is tented up to allow safe entry with scissors

Video 7 – Clamshell incision in an arrested patient

Compared to the previous videos, this demonstrates the fantastic exposure you get from the clamshell incision. This method allows the operator to quickly get into the pericardium, release the tamponade and perform two handed massage. The incision provides complete access to the heart and lungs and in this case a lung injury can easily be repaired.

Video 8 – Clamshell incision in an elective patient

The purpose of this video is to demonstrate the clamshell incision a little more slowly in an elective patient. Note that the incision in the 5th intercostal space curves up into both axillae in line with the ribs. The intercostal muscles are divided directly above the sixth rib in order to avoid damaging the neurovascular bundle and a finger is placed behind to protect the structures beneath. In the elective setting the internal mammary arteries are identified, tied and divided. In an emergency this is not required, but be aware that if output is restored these will begin to bleed and will require identifying and tying/clipping. In the elective setting a saw is used for the sternum. You can appreciate again the exposure you get from the clamshell incision with two retractors inserted. Repair of the incision is demonstrated with sutures. The incision is just a couple of centimetres below the nipples and they have curved up slightly over the sternum. In an emergency we would recommend going straight across but still aiming to curve up into both axillae.

A stressful thoracotomy

eLearning Module 4 talks through a video of a more frantic resuscitative thoracotomy, however it provides some good learning points. The patient is a motorcyclist who has sustained blunt trauma and presented without a pulse. When a patient presents in arrest like this, every second counts and working quickly and efficiently as a team is crucial.

Key learning points:
- Pause external cardiac massage whilst the thoracotomy is being performed
  - It is likely to be ineffective and will slow down the thoracotomy
- Practise and be familiar with your unit's equipment e.g. the retractor
- A clamshell incision gives the best access to the whole of the chest and allows assessment for other injuries
- There should be clear leadership and the members of the team should work well together

It is easy to comprehend how, in such a stressful scenario, the resuscitative efforts can become disorganised and chaotic. We are sure many of you have witnessed or been part of such experiences. Our hope is that by having a protocol, clear leadership structure and being well versed as a team in managing these patients, we can mitigate these risks. Given the low numbers of patients presenting in this way, the only solution is to practise in teams on mannequins. This way all members of the team will know what to do and will be able to act quickly and efficiently to ensure the best possible outcome for the patient.

RESUSCITATIVE THORACOTOMY EQUIPMENT
eLearning Module 5

It is crucial that you have the necessary equipment to perform a resuscitative thoracotomy, release a tamponade and control bleeding. At the same time, it is important not to have a large number of unnecessary instruments, making it difficult to find what you need. Learning from our own experience we have noted one of the greatest stressors during resuscitative thoracotomies is the search for instruments and disposables that may not be immediately to hand in an emergency department. This can lead to the team focussing on providing equipment rather than dealing with the patient in front of them. We strongly believe that if instrument trays are standardised across UK emergency departments, this will ensure that all clinicians know exactly what equipment is available wherever they are working.

Emergency Room Thoracotomy Sets: Resuscitative Thoracotomy 1 (RT1) and Resuscitative Thoracotomy 2 (RT2):

The first set, RT1, enables rapid initial access to the chest. It is deliberately made up separately, consisting of only a few items, to make it easily accessible and avoids the need to sift through a larger tray of instruments. The second tray, RT2, contains a greater selection of instruments including suitable equipment for emergency interventions in the emergency department. Surgical teams should be mindful that, in an emergency, a suitable suture and needle holder is perfectly adequate even if it wouldn't necessarily be their first choice in an elective theatre!

RT1 (open first)

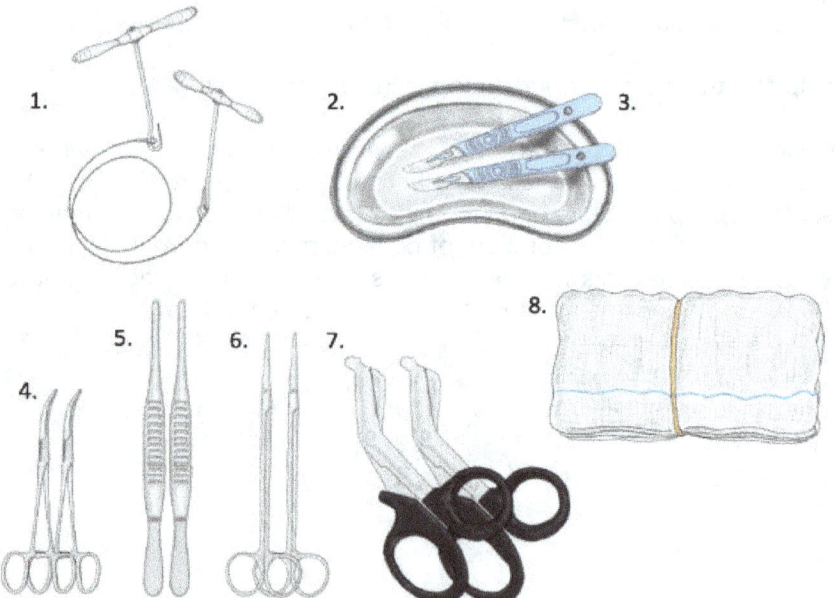

Tray RT1
1. Gigli Saw
2. Kidney dish for sharps
3. 2 Scalpels (Size 24 blades)
4. 2 x Spencer Wells artery forceps
5. 2 x Long Debakey forceps
6. 2 x Metzenbaum Scissors
7. 2 x plaster shears (dividing tissue including cutting across the sternum)
8. 5 large swabs or packs (for blood but also useful for retracting lung)

Resuscitative Thoracotomy instrument tray 1 (RT1)

This set enables two clinicians to be simultaneously performing a thoracotomy. Note depending on your local sterile services the scalpel blades may have to be separate but taped on top of the RT1 pack and the surgical nurse assistant may need to open these into the tray.

RT2 (open second)

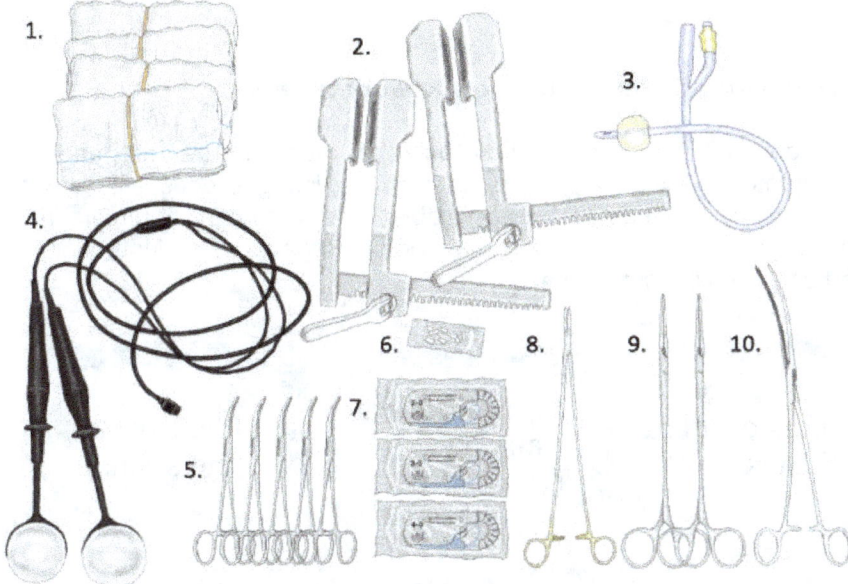

Tray RT2
1. 20x medium swabs
2. 2x Finochietto retractors
3. Foley catheter *(can be kept separate)*
4. Internal defibrillator *(alternatively external pads can be used)*
5. 5x Artery forceps
6. Teflon Pledgets
7. 5x 2/0 Prolene, 5x 3/0 Prolene, 5x 4/0 Prolene
8. Long needle holder
9. 2x Roberts forceps – *large, can be used to grasp the pericardium and, if need be, clamp vessels / other structures*
10. Long vascular clamp

Resuscitative Thoracotomy instrument tray 2 (RT2)

Other equipment

You will also require a drape for the patient. We recommend an all-in-one drape with a clear centre that can be placed onto the chest and spread to cover the rest of the patient. This also provides a sterile surface to place trays or instruments. The arms can be brought out to the side to allow ongoing access for lines/blood gases. It is not recommended to place surgical scrub solution onto the chest as it won't have time to work.

Otherwise, the equipment is the same as for any other trauma patient including rapid infusion devices e.g. the Belmont® Rapid Infuser.

WORKING AS A TEAM IN RESUSCITATIVE THORACOTOMY: THE PROTOCOL

eLearning Module 5

Practical considerations in the Emergency Department – How to work together

Centres may be using ATLS[14] or European Trauma Course[15] protocols for managing trauma patients. Our protocols are designed to be integrated with and expand on these existing processes, as well as incorporating specialist surgical teams. This needs to be applicable both in tertiary centres that have experienced cardiothoracic or trauma surgeons and in units that don't. Regardless of institution, these protocols will need to be practised and roles allocated in advance.

- An extension of ATLS
- Integrate with Surgeons
- Reproducible at any level 1 Trauma Centre
- Identify key personnel

In the remainder of this chapter, we will cover the following:

- Discussion of the indications for resuscitative thoracotomy
- Allocating roles and responsibilities
- Preparation following a pre-alert
- The variety of situations faced
- Transfer of the successfully resuscitated patient to an operating theatre

The following two chapters cover the steps of performing the resuscitative thoracotomy itself and then the time out, a key element of this protocol.

Indications

It is imperative that each institution has agreed strict criteria for those suitable for resuscitative thoracotomy, in order to avoid lengthy discussion when a patient presents in extremis.

Outcomes for blunt trauma are very poor and caution should be taken when considering resuscitative thoracotomies on these patients. However, there are no internationally agreed protocols and, as previously discussed, the ERC[1] and Eastern Association for the Surgery of Trauma[9] suggest the following indications:

- **Chest trauma with loss of output of less than 15 minutes** (survival 21% penetrating, 4.6% blunt)
- **Consider non-thoracic trauma with exsanguinating blood loss in order to clamp the descending aorta**

Furthermore, thought should be given to whether the time should be taken from loss of pulse or loss of signs of life, as the literature is variable in this regard.

Contraindications:

- Loss of cardiac output more than 15 minutes
- Patients with a cardiac output
    - Should be transferred to an operating room if possible
    - Unless too unstable - SBP<70 with evidence of tamponade (see Melbourne guidelines)
- Other injuries not compatible with life

Top tip
At the earliest opportunity, discuss within your unit your own criteria for resuscitative thoracotomy

We hope that in due course we can develop a UK wide consensus and provide stronger guidance.

Preparing to receive a patient

The following steps should be made in preparation after receiving a pre-alert from prehospital services for a patient with penetrating chest trauma:
- Trauma Team call
- Alert Cardiothoracic Surgery or locally agreed alternative surgeons
- Activate major haemorrhage protocol
    - Including rapid infusion devices
- Appropriate PPE
- Make available the Resuscitative Thoracotomy sets (RT1 and RT2)
- If high risk for ED Thoracotomy then designated operators and assistant can gown and glove prior to arrival
- Suction available
- Introductions to team in advance and assign roles
- Inform theatres (and determine where you would be going)

The Team

The team leader is responsible for allocating roles. In many institutions the use of trauma tabards or stickers is now commonplace. In the face of an unexpected trauma patient, or when multiple traumas stretch resources, there needs to be some flexibility in who is performing each role. However, in an ideal situation, we recommend the following:
- The Team Leader
- Anaesthetist
- ODP / Nurse assistant for the anaesthetist
- Doctor allocated to vascular access
- Operator (Senior ED clinician, surgeon or suitably trained physician)
- Surgical Assistant
- Surgical Nurse / health professional (scrubbed)
- Resource Coordinator

The team set-up is demonstrated in the diagram below:

The 8 key roles.
TL: Team Leader,   CO: Coordinator,   IV: Venous Access,   SN: Surgical Nurse
OP: Operating Surgeon,   AS: Surgical Assistant,   ODP: Operating Department Practitioner,   AN: Anaesthetist.

Trauma team layout for receiving a patient with traumatic chest injuries

Key protocol elements:

The following are key parts of this protocol and hence we have highlighted them here before discussing in further depth below:

- **TEAM LEADER summary of roles:**
    - Ensure allocation of roles and performance of member tasks
    - Guide all clinicians including surgeons
    - Make the decision to perform the resuscitative thoracotomy
    - Ensure active followership (including verbal feedback to the team leader at all stages from all team members)
- **RESOURCE COORDINATOR summary of roles:**
    - Coordinates equipment and major haemorrhage protocol
    - Ensures thoracotomy sets available and prepared
    - Liaises with prehospital team, theatres, surgeons
- **Arriving staff briefed and introduced to team**
- **10 minute time out - to ensure progress and coordination**
- **Staff minimisation in the resus bay**

Team leader:

It is vital that a team leader, most often the most senior emergency physician, is identified and the other key roles allocated prior to patient arrival (if possible). **All** communication should be via the team leader and if new members arrive and join the team (e.g. surgical team members), they should make themselves known to the team leader. A culture of active followership should be encouraged whereby each team member feeds back to the team leader at all stages, particularly the examination findings and any interventions made. The team leader will also guide the clinicians, including the surgeons, and make the decision about whether to perform a resuscitative thoracotomy.

Resource coordinator:

The other key concept, as part of our protocol, is the role of resource coordinator. Chest trauma patients are likely to need multiple interventions, input from several teams and onward transfer to CT or theatre. Every step is time critical and so it is vital that someone is assisting the team leader to prevent any delays. The resource coordinator is responsible for facilitating each of these stages by ensuring that the relevant equipment and personnel are available. Prior to patient arrival, they should activate the major haemorrhage protocol, arrange for rapid infusion devices and the thoracotomy sets to be available and ensure the relevant team members, including surgeons, are present. They will also need to liaise with the prehospital team, theatres, porters and CT. They need to maintain constant communication with the team leader and also ensure that a time out (described in the next chapter) occurs. A 'resource coordinator checklist' is discussed later in this chapter.

Protocol for initial management of a patient with penetrating chest trauma

NB this is designed to work in conjunction with your ATLS or ETC protocols. We summarise the initial ABC assessment and management before considering each of the team members' individual roles.

Pre-alert: Penetrating Chest Trauma – CARDIAC ARREST
- Trauma Call
- Alert Surgeons and Inform Theatres
- Activate Major Haemorrhage Protocol
- Locate Equipment: Trays, Drapes, PPE, Suction

Team Assembles
- Choose Team Leader
- Allocate Roles
- See "Key Roles" Poster

Patient Arrives ABCDE Assessment
- A. Secure Airway
- B. Apply Sats Probe, Check Trachea Central and Bilateral Air Entry. BILATERAL OPEN THORACOSTOMIES – diagnostic and therapeutic
- C. Apply ECG monitoring, NIBP, Confirm Cardiac Arrest, Obtain Vascular Access, Blood Samples, Transfuse 1:1:1 Red Cells:FFP:Platelets

PAUSE TO MAKE DECISION
- THE TEAM LEADER DECIDES IF CRITERIA ARE MET TO PERFORM EMERGENCY RESUSCITATIVE THORACOTOMY
- "Is the Airway Secured?"
- "Is there Vascular Access?"
- "Is the Surgical Team Scrubbed and is RT1 Open and Ready to Use with Suction Available?"

"PERFORM RESUSCITATIVE THORACOTOMY"

Anaesthetist

SECURE AIRWAY

Obtain Vascular access

- Peripheral cannula / central access / intraosseous
- If it is not possible to obtain access, then the team leader needs to communicate with the surgeons to obtain access from within the chest e.g. a cannula into the right atrium
- Manage infusions and transfusions

ODP

ASSIST THE ANAESTHETIST

- Secure the airway
- Prepare for Rapid Sequence Induction
- Prepare sedation and muscle paralysis

Assist in obtaining vascular access

- Manage infusions and transfusions
- Send off crossmatch, blood gas, bloods

Vascular access doctor

ESTABLISH VENOUS ACCESS

- Large Bore Venous Access
- Central venous Access / Intraosseous Access
- Escalate to team leader if concerns - direct right atrial access can be a last resort

Blood samples

- Crossmatch (twice),
- Blood gas (arterial or venous)
- FBC, U&E, Clotting

Operator

Take commands from Team Leader

Lead Clamshell Thoracotomy

- Open by bilateral thoracostomies, extended to thoracotomy
- Join opposite thoracotomy across the lower sternum or xiphisternum

Once Clamshell performed

- Open pericardium medial but parallel to the phrenic nerve
- Suction blood
- Look for site of bleeding
- Consider clamping/compressing the descending aorta (if output restored)
  NB no point clamping aorta if no output. If in VF focus on shocking. If internal massage required and heart empty then really filling is key.

Surgical Assistant

Assist operator with the Clamshell

- Perform thoracostomy
- Extend this into thoracotomies
- Assist operator completing cut across the sternum
- Retract the sternum cranially
- Insert Finochietto retractors
- Assist operator with suction, lung retraction, bleeding control

Nurse assistant / Surgical nurse

Prior to the Resuscitative Thoracotomy

- Don Gown and Gloves
- Open RT1 surgical instruments and drapes
- Open Yankauer sucker and have it connected to high suction
- Lay out instruments for thoracotomy and hand in order below

Order of instruments

- Drape (preferably all in one with transparent centre)
    NB it is not recommended to prep the skin in these patients
- Scalpels
- Scissors
- Plaster shears or Gigli saw for sternum
- Finochietto retractors
- Sucker, packs and be ready to open RT2

Resource coordinator

Team Preparation

- Ensure correct personnel are in the resuscitation room
- Ensure Thoracotomy sets RT1 and RT2 are available
- Ensure Operating Theatre is aware
- Ensure Blood Transfusion are aware
- Act as the team scribe
- Complete resource coordinator checklist

Interaction with Team Leader

- May need to prepare for transfer to the operating room
- May need further surgical equipment (Diathermy, cell salvage)
- May need laparotomy
- May need REBOA

Resource coordinator checklist:

CATEGORY	ACTION	Y/N
INITIAL	**Ensure all positions allocated by Team Leader** Direct arriving staff to Team Leader	
	Activate Major Haemorrhage Protocol	
	Request Surgeons attend	
	Inform Theatre Team to prepare +/- attend	
	Confirm surgical equipment arrives: Resuscitative Thoracotomy Trays RT1 & RT2 Drape, Gowns, Gloves Defibrillator with internal paddle function Suction	
	Ensure posters up: Key Roles Key Equipment	
	Set timer once patient arrives/ Note key events	
DURING	**Liaise / Update External Teams:** Blood Services/ Transfusion Labs for investigations Radiology Theatre Team Other Teams as required	
	At 10 mins inform Team Lead to do Time Out	
	Direct arriving staff to Team Leader If required (keep numbers in resus low) Ensure presence announced/ team aware	
NEAR CLOSE	**Plan for patient transfer/ Theatre Checklist**	
	Ensure Team Leader's De-Brief & Notes completed	

Note that the checklist can be amended to suit individual institution requirements.

> **Top tip**
> **Print physical copies of the checklist or have the flip chart to be used at each chest trauma resuscitation**

Summary

This chapter has summarised the key roles, the equipment required, relevant checklists and a protocol for preparation and initial management of these patients. The next two chapters cover the resuscitative thoracotomy itself followed by the 'time out' and remainder of the protocol. These are clearly complex scenarios demanding a lot of concurrent activity. By practising simulations within your institution you can become skilled as a team, your resuscitative thoracotomies will become well organised and this will translate into better patient outcomes.

PERFORMING THE RESUSCITATIVE THORACOTOMY

eLearning Module 6

Surgical approaches to the chest:

There are several approaches to the chest depending on the scenario:

- **'Clamshell'**
- Alternatives are
    - **Left thoracotomy**
    - **Sternotomy**

Our strong advice is that a clamshell should be performed for all patients who require emergency access to the chest in the emergency department, or indeed in the prehospital setting. We have seen in previous chapters the difficulty faced due to limited access through a single thoracotomy. If the patient is stable enough for transfer to theatre, then a specialist surgeon can consider a thoracotomy or sternotomy as an alternative. The latter procedure requires a specialist saw and is most suitable for more central injuries. Cardiothoracic surgeons are more familiar with working through this incision, however, we do not recommend it to be performed in the emergency department. If the indication is thought to be solely to allow clamping of the aorta for an extra-thoracic injury then a left thoracotomy could be performed initially.

The Resuscitative 'Clamshell' Thoracotomy

As previously mentioned, this course is not designed to teach the procedure itself in any great depth. We would urge you to attend specific cadaveric or other wet lab courses to gain this experience. The following are the key steps in performing a resuscitative 'clamshell' thoracotomy followed by some tips regarding interventions within the chest.

1. Open RT1 tray

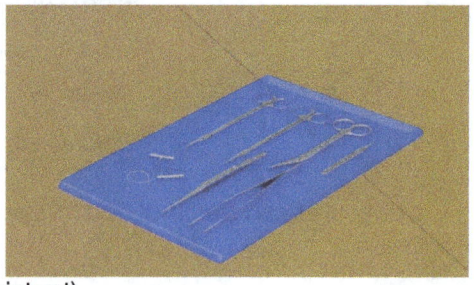

2. Gown and glove (minimum 2 operators and one assistant)

3. Lie the patient flat with their arms preferably at 90 degrees

4. Apply an all-in-one drape across the patient

5. Assess where your clamshell incision will be; roughly 2cm under the nipples, curved upwards laterally to the mid axillary line, aiming for the 5th intercostal space

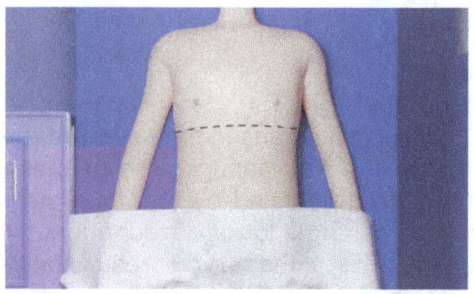

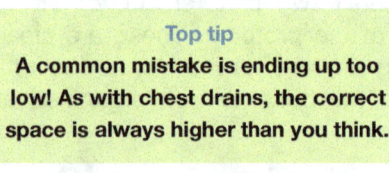

Top tip
A common mistake is ending up too low! As with chest drains, the correct space is always higher than you think.

6. Using the scalpel, start by making bilateral thoracostomies and place a finger into the chest, looking for evidence of tension pneumothorax (large hiss of air, lung down) or haemothorax. Reassess the patient to see if output is restored. If no output, proceed to step 7.

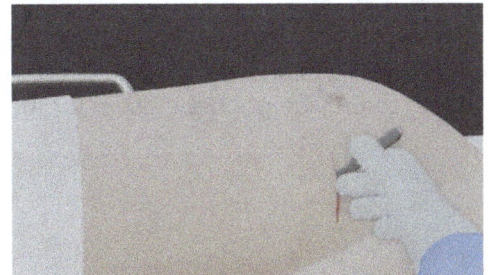

7. Both the operators should then extend their respective incisions on each side to the midline using a scalpel to cut through the tissue until the ribs and intercostal spaces are visible

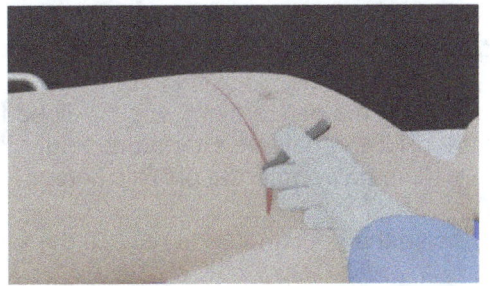

8. Using scissors to avoid damaging the lung beneath, cut through the intercostal muscles

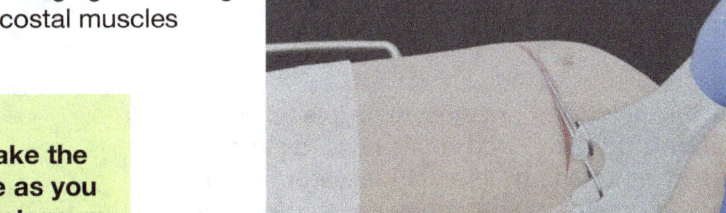

Top tip

Exposure is key so make the thoracotomies as large as you can - all the way to the sternum and posteriorly as far as you can.

9. Cut horizontally across the sternum using the heavy plaster shears to complete the clamshell

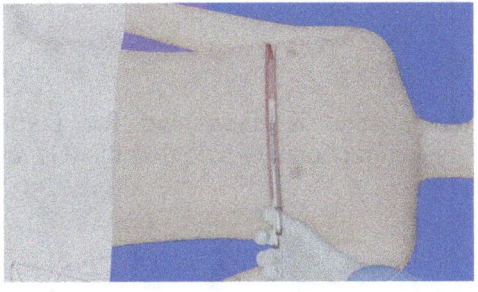

- If this is too difficult then either:
    - Use a Gigli saw by passing an instrument immediately behind the sternum and pulling the saw through
      OR
    - Cut inferiorly on both sides along the sternal edge using the shears to a point where you can cut across the sternum or xiphisternum

10. Using two hands the assistant retracts the clamshell, preferably from above the patient's head, to provide good exposure for the operator

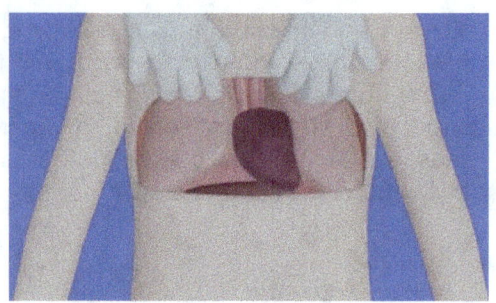

From this stage onwards the exact steps now vary depending on the clinical findings.

11. Pick up the pericardium, which will be tense with blood if the patient is tamponading, close to the midline away from the phrenic nerves

12. Incise the pericardium to release the tamponade

13. Extend the incision to enable the heart to be delivered for further examination and internal massage if required

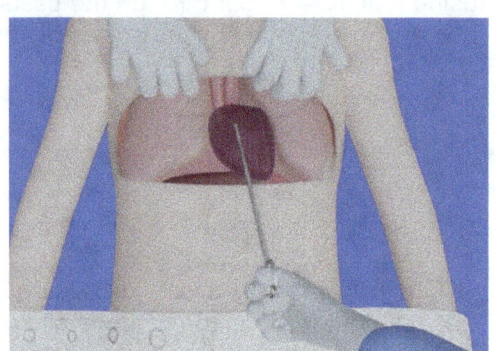

14. If the heart has arrested, then place one hand behind the heart and a flat hand on top of the heart and perform internal massage taking care not to press the tips of any digits into the heart muscle

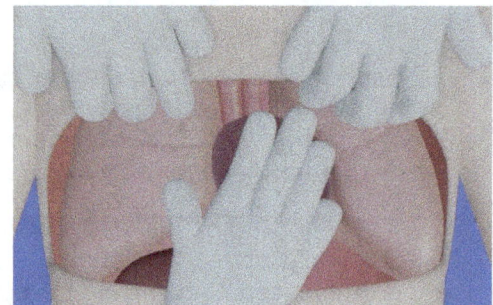

15. Whilst this is happening the surgical nurse assistant should ensure that the RT2 tray is open

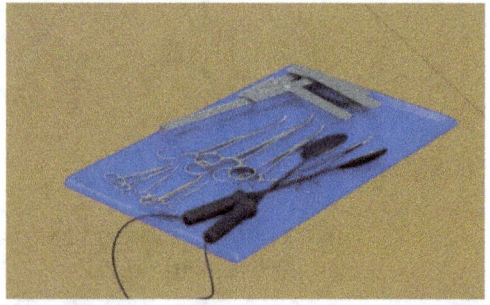

16. Insert Finochietto retractors and open as widely as possible

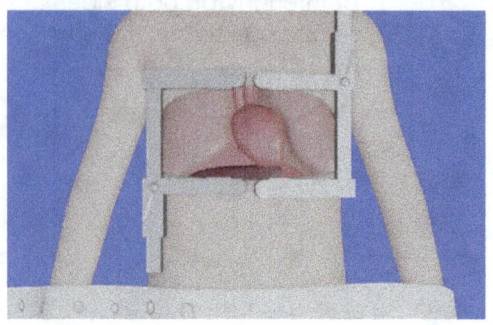

17. Further management will depend on the injuries encountered however you should now have enough exposure and the relevant equipment to deal with injuries to the thoracic structures

18. If the patient arrests and is in a shockable rhythm then internal defibrillator paddles should be used. If not available, close the clamshell and shock with external pads.

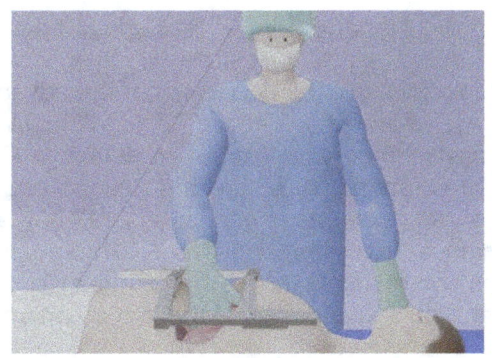

19. Throughout the procedure, feedback to the team leader your findings and any interventions performed

Internal cardiac massage

Video 2 in *eLearning module 3a* demonstrates the technique of internal cardiac massage. Before attempting internal massage, fully 'deliver' the heart through the open pericardium, inspect the heart and try to remove any blood clots that you see. Pass the right hand over the apex of the heart and then advance further around the apex to the back of the heart, palm up and hand flat. The left hand is then placed flat onto the anterior surface of the heart and the two hands squeezed together. Flat palms and straight fingers are important to avoid an unequal distribution of pressure onto the heart, thereby minimising the chance of trauma. In particular never dip your thumb into the heart as it can tear. The right ventricle is particularly fragile if it is distended during an arrest. Be mindful to keep the heart as horizontal as possible and not lift it vertically, as this can obstruct flow. Squeeze your hands together at a rate of 100bpm and, if an arterial line is present, look at the trace to verify adequate internal massage. You should try to obtain a systolic impulse of more than 60mmHg.

Internal defibrillator paddles

During the course we will demonstrate how to use the internal defibrillator paddles. These should be part of your RT2 instrument tray and you must ensure that they are compatible with the defibrillator in your resus bays. The operator, assistant or surgical nurse should pass the end of the lead to a non-scrubbed team member to connect to the defibrillator.

Internal defibrillator paddles are a more effective way of applying current directly to the heart and hence much lower energy levels are selected. The paddles are placed within the pericardium either side of the heart; one over the right atrium/ventricle and the other over the apex. The defibrillator should be charged to 20J and the shock is administered either by pressing and holding the button on the top of the defibrillator paddle or from the defibrillator itself, depending on the model.

If you don't have internal defibrillator paddles, then external pads can still be used but you must close the clamshell incision for them to be effective. Remember that team members should also all be clear and not touching the patient or trolley.

Advanced management of thoracic injuries

The main focus of the course is not the advanced techniques required for definitive management of these patients, which often requires a cardiothoracic theatre team after transfer to a theatre with access to specialist equipment. Video 4 in *eLearning module 3b* demonstrates how difficult it can be, even for cardiac surgeons, to suture the beating heart. In the resus environment simple manoeuvres can often suffice, for example digital pressure, however we will briefly outline some of the more advanced techniques that can be used by more experience practitioners. Instrument tray RT2 contains the equipment required for the techniques described. This section is aimed at surgeons or operators with relevant training and experience, but others may find it interesting nevertheless.

Cardiac/great vessel injuries

As mentioned above, it is vital that the pericardium is opened fully to allow thorough inspection for injuries and access for further intervention. Evacuate any blood or clots using suction and your fingers. If tamponade was the aetiology of the arrest then this in itself may restore cardiac output, but be prepared for any wounds to now start bleeding profusely. If the heart is in asystole then attempt to flick the ventricle reasonably firmly as this can restore the rhythm or, if not, then commence internal massage as described above. If the heart is in a shockable rhythm, then internal defibrillation should be performed. Attention must now be turned to management of any traumatic wounds.

Surgical bleeding can often be controlled with direct digital pressure,[16] particularly if the wound is small. Swabs/gauze can also be used to pack bleeding points or be pressed firmly against structures with the operator's fingers. If this is enough to control bleeding, then we would not advocate attempting more advanced closure unless the operator is experienced and haemodynamic stability is achieved.

Larger wounds that aren't controlled by digital pressure require more complex techniques[16,17]. A Foley catheter can be carefully inserted into larger wounds, the balloon inflated and gentle traction applied. Do not aim to fully stop bleeding in this way, as excess force can cause the balloon to enlarge the defect. As a last resort, the wound can be sutured. For ventricular wounds, place horizontal mattress sutures using Teflon pledgeted Prolene sutures.[16,17] This technique distributes the tension to prevent further tearing of the myocardium. Suture bites must also be of a reasonable depth to prevent the suture from tearing through. If Teflon pledgets are not available, they can be fashioned from small sections of pericardium. If the injury is adjacent to a coronary vessel, then caution is required to prevent occlusion of the vessel, particularly if proximal. Horizontal mattress sutures are placed with the needle passing beneath the vessel (see diagram 'Repair 3'). The external suture and knot should lie parallel, either side of the vessel and wound. An alternative to suturing ventricular injuries is using a skin stapler directly on the myocardium.

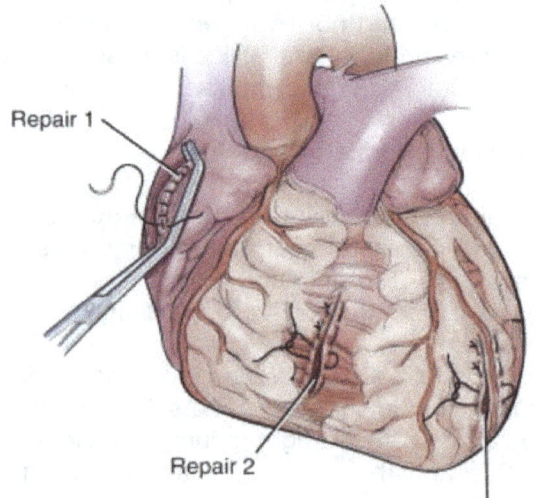

Diagram showing continuous suture technique for atrial injury *(Repair 1)*, interrupted horizontal mattress sutures for a ventricular injury *(Repair 2)* and repair of an injury adjacent to a coronary artery *(Repair 3)*. (Feliciano DV. *Rich's Vascular Trauma 2016; p76*)[16]

For atrial injuries a clamp can be placed across the hole. The injury can be subsequently sutured using a continuous technique (see diagram 'Repair 1').[16]

Posterior heart injuries should not be missed and should be suspected if the bleeding point is not immediately obvious. Management may require careful lifting of the heart, but this should be minimised and performed for short periods only, as it will interrupt venous return.[16,17] If the blood pressure is very low and the patient under-filled, this manoeuvre risks air being entrained into the heart. In this instance, examination should be limited to feeling behind the heart, occluding any hole with a finger and waiting until the patient has been further resuscitated before further examination.[16]

Finally, for large cardiac or vessel injuries causing exsanguinating bleeding in a beating heart, it may be necessary to temporarily occlude venous return to allow repair. An alternative strategy described in the literature is to give adenosine to cause temporary asystole.[16] Neither should be attempted in those without adequate training or experience.

Pulmonary/hilar injuries

Injuries to the lung can be more complex to repair as lung tissue is incredibly fragile. The majority of small peripheral injuries can be controlled with pressure or packing with swabs until definitive management, for example with thoracic surgical staplers, can be performed. Small air leaks from lung tissue are not going to cause the patient harm and with the chest open the risk of tension pneumothorax is eliminated. For larger peripheral injuries suturing can be attempted or alternatively the aortic cross clamp can be placed across the tissue[16] until the arrival of a thoracic surgeon.

Proximal or hilar injuries are more difficult to manage. Smaller injuries may be managed with pressure or packing. If there are large defects, then massive haemorrhage may occur and there is a risk of fatal systemic air embolism (discussed further in the 'Special circumstances in thoracic trauma' chapter). These injuries require emergency techniques as temporising measures before definitive thoracic surgical intervention. There are several methods to occlude the hilar structures,[16,18] but the inferior pulmonary ligament must be divided first for these to be effective. Initially a hand can be placed around the hilum, grasping firmly. Subsequently, the most straightforward method is to place a large clamp across the hilum, however, rigidity of the bronchus may prevent complete vascular control. An alternative method is to encircle the hilum with the Foley catheter or a tie, snaring/tourniqueting the hilar structures. The catheter/tie is secured with a clamp. Finally, another recognised method is the hilar twist where the lung is rotated 180 degrees.[16,18] The benefit of this method is that it does not require any specialist equipment or training, however this should be done carefully to prevent tearing vessels further. If the injury extends more proximally to within the pericardium, then these methods may not provide adequate control. In this instance, it is necessary to approach the vessels from within the pericardium and place vascular clamps.

Other techniques that limit air embolism include avoiding high inflation pressures and single lung ventilation of the 'good' lung.

Other considerations

After initial inspection of the heart, great vessels and hila, one must examine the whole of the thorax for signs of trauma. The benefit of the clamshell incision is that it provides fantastic exposure of the majority of the chest. In the case of penetrating trauma, the entry point is an obvious place to start. Injury to the intercostal neurovascular bundles can cause significant haemorrhage over time but is easily controlled with pressure or clips. Other areas to assess include structures at the thoracic inlet and the descending aorta. Finally, after output is restored the clamshell incision will begin to bleed. At this stage, the only real concern is any bleeding arteries in the chest wall and the internal mammary vessels. These can also be temporarily controlled with clips.

We have already discussed the uses of the Foley catheter as a method of controlling bleeding from the heart and snaring the hilum. A third function is to give blood products.[17] If the catheter has been inserted into the heart through a defect, then blood products can be given directly into the atria or ventricles. This is particularly useful if vascular access has not been secured and, given the large calibre of the catheter, large volumes can be infused rapidly.

Summary

This chapter has described step by step how to perform the resuscitative 'clamshell' thoracotomy. Internal cardiac massage and defibrillation has also been discussed. It is important that all team members, and not just the operators or surgeons, are aware of these procedures to ensure that there is a common understanding of what to expect during these resuscitations. This enables the team to work more effectively and allows all team members to contribute or highlight issues. The latter section of the chapter considered more advanced techniques of managing thoracic injuries. These should only be attempted by those with relevant training or experience and teaching these techniques is not the aim of this course.

THE TIME OUT AND BEYOND IN RESUSCITATIVE THORACOTOMY
eLearning Module 6

We would like to introduce an important concept into this resuscitative thoracotomy protocol, which is the performance of a **time out**. This should be carried out either when there is a period of stability, perhaps after the chest has been opened and bleeding is controlled, or after 10 minutes of resuscitation. The team leader then calls for a **time out** to assess the current situation. We advise using the acronym **TRAUMATIC CROSS** (see below).

Ideally this would be physically written on a handheld flip chart, wall poster or crib sheet and could even be placed as a tick sheet on top of your resuscitative thoracotomy packs. The **TRAUMATIC** acronym was initially developed in one of our centres for any bleeding major trauma patient[19] and we feel it applies particularly well to patients who have sustained chest injuries. The management principles should be thought about throughout the whole resuscitation, however, the last column of each table highlights some crucial points to think about during the time out.

	RESUSCITIVE THORACOTOMY = TRAUMATIC CROSS		TIME OUT @ 10 minutes
T	**Tranexamic Acid**	- Initial 1g bolus: • Often already given pre-hospital • Otherwise, administer only if within 3 hours of injury or ongoing hyperfibrinolysis • Do not delay, every minute counts - Subsequent 1g infusion over 8 hours	- Has first TXA been given?
R	**Resuscitation**	- Activate Major Haemorrhage Protocol - Initial Transfusion Ratio 1:1:1 and consider: • Rapid infuser and cell salvage • Time-limited hypotensive resuscitation • Pelvic binder / splint fractures / tourniquet - Avoid any crystalloid use	- Assess how well we have managed to resuscitate the patient • What is the BP? HR? • How much volume have we given? and what? (1:1:1) • Is heart well filled? - Further blood products required? - A-line? Urinary catheter?
A	**Avoid Hypothermia**	- Target temperature > 36°C • Increase ambient theatre temperature • Remove wet clothing and sheets • Warm all blood products & irrigation fluids • Warm the patient using forced-air warming device / blanket / mattress	- Adequate temperature probe e.g. oral - Document temperature - Warming adjuncts in place - Prevent cooling
U	**Unstable? Damage Control Surgery**	- If unstable, coagulopathic, hypothermic or acidotic, perform damage control surgery of: • Haemorrhage control, decompression, decontamination and splintage - Time surgery aiming to finish < 90mins and conduct Surgical Pauses at least every 30mins	- Straight to theatre now? - Possibility of injuries elsewhere? • Does the patient require involvement of other surgical teams e.g. requires laparotomy
M	**Metabolic**	- Perform regular blood gas analysis - Base excess and lactate guide resuscitation • Adequate resuscitation corrects acidosis - If lactate > 5mmol/L or rising, consider stopping surgery, splint and transfer to ICU - Haemoglobin results are misleading	- Check the blood gas - What is their metabolic status? - Are the gases improving?
A	**Avoid Vasoconstrictors**	- Use of vasoconstrictors doubles mortality • However, use may be required in cases of spinal cord or traumatic brain injury - Anaesthetic induction -Suggest Ketamine - Maintenance -When BP allows, titrate high dose Fentanyl and consider Midazolam	- Volume or vasopressor indicated? - If heart well filled and poorly contractile consider inotropes
T	**Test Clotting**	- Check clotting regularly to target transfusion: • Laboratory or point of care (TEG / ROTEM) - Aim platelets > 100x10^9/L - Aim INR & aPTTR ≤ 1.5 - Aim fibrinogen > 2g/L	- Bloods sent?
I	**Imaging**	- Consider: • CT: Most severely injured / haemodynamically unstable patients gain most from CT • Interventional radiology	- Can we get to CT? - eFAST results?
C	**Calcium**	- Maintain ionised Calcium > 1.0 mmol/L • Administer 10mls of 10% Calcium Chloride over 10 minutes, repeating as required - Monitor Potassium and treat hyperkalaemia with Calcium and Insulin/Glucose	- Check blood gas? - Give calcium?

Adapted from "Major Trauma? Major Haemorrhage?" guideline 2019 University Hospitals Coventry and Warwickshire NHS Trust

		TIME OUT @ 10 MINUTES
C	Cause	- What was the cause of the arrest? • Any extra-thoracic injuries causing hypovolaemia? - What injuries have we found? • Isolated chest? other injuries?
R	ROSC?	- Have we got a return of spontaneous circulation?
O	Open	- Is the surgical access sufficient to assess and control all bleeding? • Extend excision / improve retraction
S S S	Surgically Salvageable?	- Can bleeding be controlled? - Are the injuries repairable? - Is this injury survivable?

The time out should allow the team to assess exactly where they are in terms of resuscitating the patient, gauge how well the patient is responding to interventions and ensure that critical steps or treatments haven't been omitted. We would suggest silence in the room during this process if possible.

The time out also provides an opportunity for the team leader to think about whether we need additional expert help. For example, if there is concern about bleeding in the abdomen or pelvis, have the general surgeons or orthopaedics been contacted? Could the patient benefit from REBOA? Are there any further investigations required? Consult all team members; the anaesthetist may want a CXR to confirm line or tube placement before moving on. If it is clear that the injuries found are not salvageable an early decision should be made to stop further resuscitation/surgery.

Where will the patient be transferred to next?

Guided by the TRAUMATIC CROSS assessment, a discussion will be necessary about where to go from the resus bay. Most likely, this will be a decision about going to CT or to theatre depending on stability. Either way, before any patient transfer, we advise a checklist to be performed to ensure that the patient is transferred safely and with the necessary equipment.

> **Transfer to theatre checklist**
> ✓ Is the bleeding controlled? (transfers can be 5-10 minutes)
> ✓ Is the theatre ready to receive the patient?
> ✓ Are any other procedures needed in the ED?
>   – Central line, arterial line, ET Tube, Laparotomy?
> ✓ Place packs in the chest, remove retractors and cover the wound
> ✓ Check for other sources of bleeding e.g. internal mammary arteries which may benefit from the placement of a clip
> ✓ If an airtight dressing is used to cover the wound, insert a chest drain (even just under the dressing) to prevent a tension pneumothorax
> ✓ Obtain mobile monitoring and a portable ventilator
> ✓ Team leader: brief team on transfer plan including plan for lifts and plan if the patient becomes unstable

NON-ARREST SITUATIONS IN PENETRATING THORACIC TRAUMA

eLearning Module 7

This module explores the management of patients presenting with penetrating chest injuries but who have not arrested. Your approach should be as per your ATLS[14] or European Trauma Course protocols,[15] as you would with any other trauma patients. However, we will touch on some of the important management principles for this subgroup of patients.

It is important to remember the possible aetiology of peri-arrest situations in penetrating thoracic trauma. We suggest using the acronym HOTT:

- **H**ypovolaemia
- **O**xygenation
- **T**ension pneumothorax
- **T**amponade

The major issues to exclude early on in a patient who still has an output following chest trauma are the last two and should be actively looked for during your primary survey. The fact that these patients have an output obviously means that you have a little more time on your hands than those considered in the last chapter. However, this time should be used efficiently, as these patients can deteriorate rapidly. Immediate, rapid assessment is warranted and relevant team members and equipment can be assembled in anticipation of procedures or interventions.

ABCDE assessment and initial management

A suitably qualified doctor should carry out the initial ABCDE assessment according to ATLS or ETC protocols. It is not the purpose of this course to cover this in detail. Indeed, this is described well in the relevant course handbooks.[14,15] However, during the assessment of a patient with penetrating chest injuries, particular attention should be paid to ruling out the injuries discussed in the table on the following page. Relevant interventions are also given in the adjoining column. We subsequently describe the management of hypovolaemia and tamponade in greater detail.

	Assess for signs of:	Interventions:
AIRWAY	- Airways obstruction	- High flow oxygen via non-rebreathe mask (for all patients) - Airway adjuncts as appropriate: • NP, OP, LMA, ETT • Consider early surgical cricothyrodotomy if severe facial injuries
BREATHING *Consider also tracheobronchial injuries*	- Tension pneumothorax	- Needle decompression with venflon but preferably TUBE THORACOSTOMY in the triangle of safety: • Spontaneously breathing patient : Tube Thoracostomy • Intubated patient : Open Thoracostomy • Perform on the side most likely to be abnormal • Perform this on the other side if no improvement
	- Open chest wound (simple pneumothorax)	- Dressing taped on 3 sides or specialist dressings with one way valves if available - Consider chest drain, but not normally required immediately
	- Massive haemothorax	- Tube thoracostomy for monitoring • >1L will likely need intervention • >1.5-2L likely needs resuscitative thoracotomy
	- Large flail segment	- Consider early intubation or NIV if respiratory distress
CIRCULATION *Include eFAST USS specifically to look for pericardial effusion / tamponade*	Hypovolaemia from: - Cardiac Tamponade - Myocardial laceration - Pulmonary haemorrhage - Aortic Injury - Superior mediastinal vascular injury	- Large Bore IV access • Peripheral / femoral / subclavian / IO - Aggressive volume resuscitation • Transfusion as per 1:1:1 protocol - Transfusion Goals (in absence of A line) • Conscious Patient : Any signs of life • Unconscious Patient : Central pulse - Invasive arterial monitoring - If suspected, these patients need to go to theatre
DISABILITY	Reduced GCS - Primary brain injury - Secondary to hypoperfusion	Consider early imaging if stable enough • May inform decisions regarding ongoing resuscitation
EXPOSURE	Assess for injuries to the back and other compartments	Consider eFAST / CT or involvement of other teams Consider oesophageal injury

> **Top tips**
> **Tube thoracostomy**
> • Use the biggest chest drain available
> • Blunt dissection technique
> • Finger sweep to assess the lung and the presence of adhesions before drain insertion

Rapid Sequence Induction

To prevent haemodynamic collapse, avoid induction of anaesthesia if possible until tension pneumothorax or tamponade are excluded/treated. If unavoidable, ensure the surgical team is scrubbed and by the patient.

Hypovolaemia suspected:

- Transfusion as per 1:1:1 RBCs:FFP:platelets protocol
- Tranexamic acid
- Transfusion goals :
    - Conscious Patient : Any signs of life
    - Unconscious patient : Central pulse
- Avoid vasoactive drugs
    - If at all possible!
- Avoid hypothermia and replace calcium
- Consider CT scan (Thorax/Abdo/Pelvis)
- Surgical treatment in theatre or, if unstable, clamshell in the emergency department
- Consider Zone 1 REBOA if locally available

Tamponade suspected:

- Judicious resuscitation with 1:1:1 RBCs:FFP:platelets
- Guide management with eFAST findings
- If tamponade suspected in isolation then limit the volume transfused as the primary problem is compression/obstruction and not hypovolaemia
- Careful use of vasoactive agents to improve cardiac output
- Surgical treatment preferably in theatres or, if unstable, clamshell in the emergency department
- Consider USS guided pericardiocentesis (if appropriately skilled) only to buy time for expert assistance to become available

Stability

One of the hardest management decisions for a team looking after non-arrest patients with penetrating chest trauma is deciding when they are stable enough for onward transfer. Stability is the ability to stop rapid IV resuscitation for a period long enough to allow investigation without gross haemodynamic or respiratory depression. Even with CT scanners located in emergency departments, it is a 5-10 minute process at best to get the patient through the scanner. Transfers to theatre may take even longer however, for these patients, that is often where they need to be for definitive management. Although CT imaging is useful to guide surgical intervention, if a patient is not stable enough then they need to go to theatre as soon as possible. In patients in which stability has not yet been achieved then the theatre team will have to come to resus. A suggested algorithm for deciding where to transfer is:

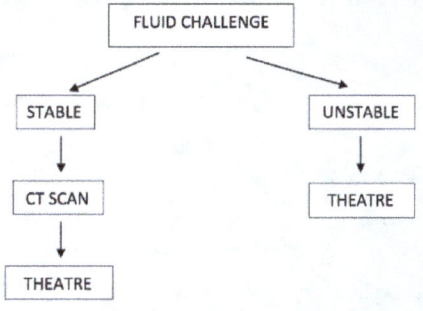

Surgical approaches in theatre

- Midline penetrating injuries: **Median Sternotomy**
    - Allows good exposure to heart and major vessels
    - Allows reasonable exposure to lung hila and is familiar to cardiac surgeons
- Lateral penetrating injury : **Thoracotomy**
    - Allows excellent exposure to hila, pulmonary artery and vein and the descending aorta on the left
    - Reasonable access to the heart

Summary

This is a very different patient group to the arrested patient. In many ways these patients are more difficult to manage as there are a plethora of possible diagnoses and consequently many more management decisions to make rather than simply proceeding to a resuscitative thoracotomy. However, if the team approach the patient with a structured ABCDE assessment, perform relevant interventions, obtain wide bore access and commence appropriate resuscitation, then this will buy time to ascertain the likely diagnosis and proceed to definitive management.

SPECIAL CIRCUMSTANCES IN THORACIC TRAUMA
eLearning Module 8

The main focus of this course is arrest and non-arrest situations in patients with chest trauma. However, given this is a course delivered in part by cardiothoracic surgeons, we felt it only right to discuss some special circumstances that we rarely see in thoracic trauma but are really quite important.

The Difficult Airway

Any major trauma, particularly those with significant facial or neck injuries, increases the risk of a difficult airway and requires input from anaesthetists who are skilled in advanced airway techniques. Assessment of the trauma patient begins with examination and management of the airway. It is likely that airway support will be necessary and therefore identifying a difficult airway is key. An individualised airway management plan for each patient should be formed in communication with members of the trauma team to ensure maximum safety and success. The Difficult Airway Society provides clear guidelines for the management of these situations[20] and should be followed.

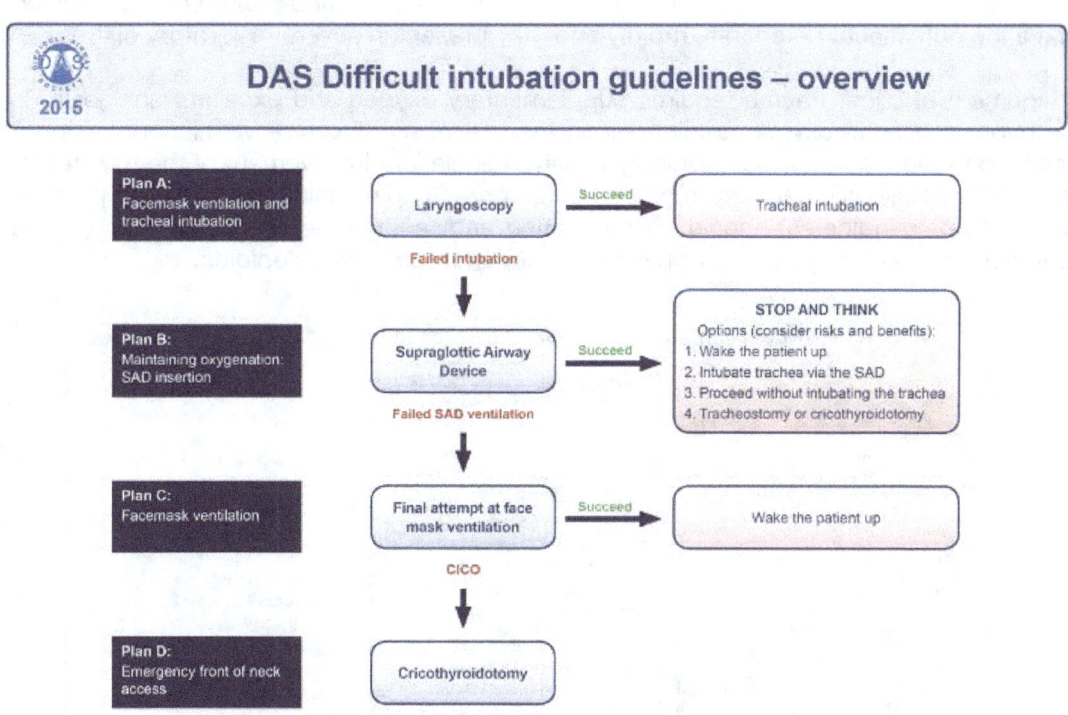

Difficult Airway Society Flowchart for Unanticipated Difficult Intubation[20]

In patients that require endotracheal intubation it is important to remember that adequate oxygenation should be achieved throughout. All patients should receive 100% oxygen, and in patients displaying signs of airway obstruction simple manoeuvres including a chin lift or jaw thrust can help to open the airway and facilitate oxygenation. The use of oropharyngeal, nasopharyngeal and supraglottic airway devices can also help to maintain the patient's airway while awaiting intubation.

In patients with injuries that prevent conventional endotracheal intubation, if immediate airway intervention is required then perform a surgical cricothyroidotomy. However, if time allows, then communication with the thoracic or ENT team is required as a tracheostomy may be the safest option.

Breathing Problems

As discussed previously, the most likely major thoracic injuries that you will encounter, and hence should be assessing for, are:
- Tension pneumothorax
- Open chest wound
- Massive haemothorax
- Large flail segment

Flail chest

Blunt trauma, for example crush injuries or RTCs, can result in significant chest injuries with multiple rib fractures and flail segments. Such significant bony injuries are, unsurprisingly, often accompanied by underlying damage to thoracic organs including lung lacerations and pulmonary contusions. These patients have the potential to deteriorate rapidly and may present in severe respiratory distress.

Initial management of chest trauma requires supplementary oxygen and excellent analgesia. In patients developing hypoxia despite oxygen administration the use of non-invasive ventilation or high flow nasal oxygen can help to reduce the risk of requiring invasive ventilation. Involvement of the pain team early and use of a rib fracture analgesia pathway improves outcomes. Simple analgesics including paracetamol and ibuprofen (if not contraindicated) should be prescribed and regional nerve catheter techniques such as serratus anterior and erector spinae nerve blocks are superior to systemic opioids.

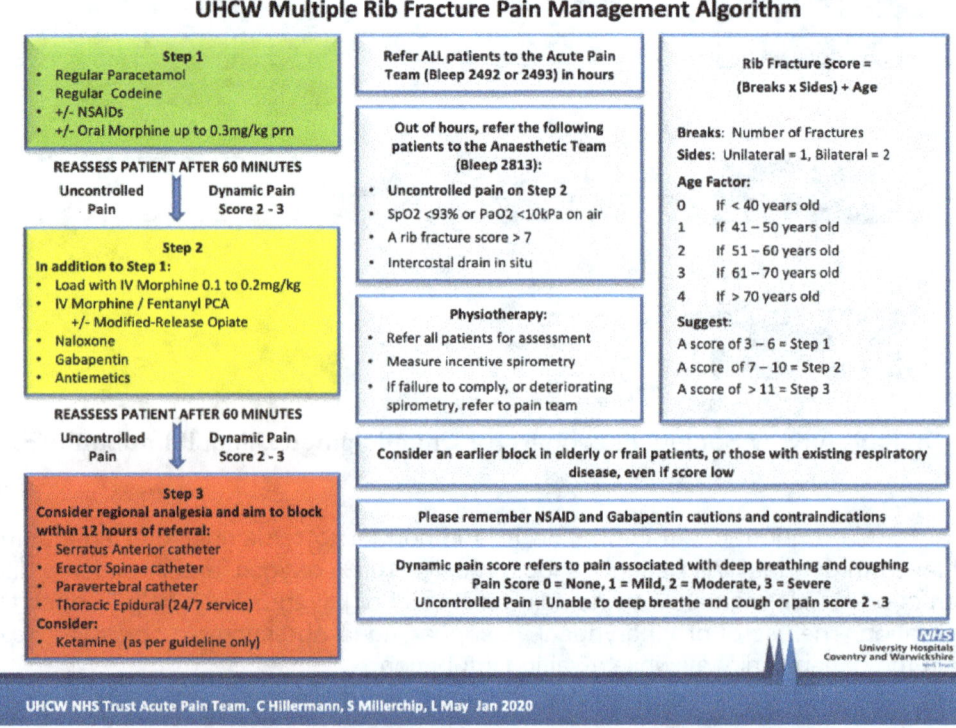

Example rib fracture pain management algorithm from UHCW[21]

With extensive flail segments, the combination of pain, altered mechanics, atelectasis, contusions and increased dead space may make self-ventilation ineffective and necessitate intubation and ventilation. Following stabilisation and initial recovery from their injuries, these patients often require rib plating to allow weaning from the ventilator or for pain management. The chest x-ray below shows a trauma patient following such a procedure. Note also that the left clavicle has been plated. The patient went on to make a very good recovery.

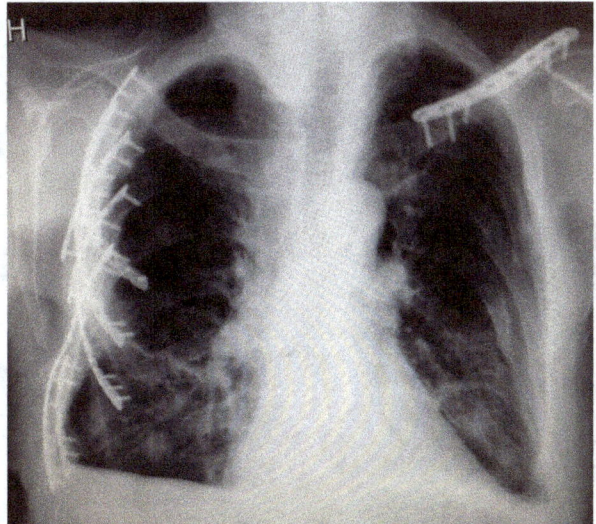

CXR of a patient post rib plating for a flail chest following a traumatic crush injury

Miscellaneous:

Aortic disruption

Aortic disruption injuries are difficult to diagnose. Aortic transection is classically associated with deceleration injuries. The heart and the arch of the aorta are more mobile in the chest, whereas the descending aorta is more fixed posteriorly. During rapid deceleration the more mobile structures are displaced anteriorly and a tear can occur just beyond the left subclavian artery at the proximal descending aorta. Complete transection is fatal and these patients die at the scene. If the aortic adventitia (outer layer) contains the injury, then these patients have a chance of surviving to hospital. However, without subsequent intervention their prognosis remains poor.

Indicators of aortic injury are:
- Widening of the superior mediastinum to >8cm
- Depression of the left main bronchus to <40° with the trachea
- Tracheal shift to the right
- Blurring of aortic outline
- Pleural cap
- Lateral displacement of the nasogastric tube in the oesophagus

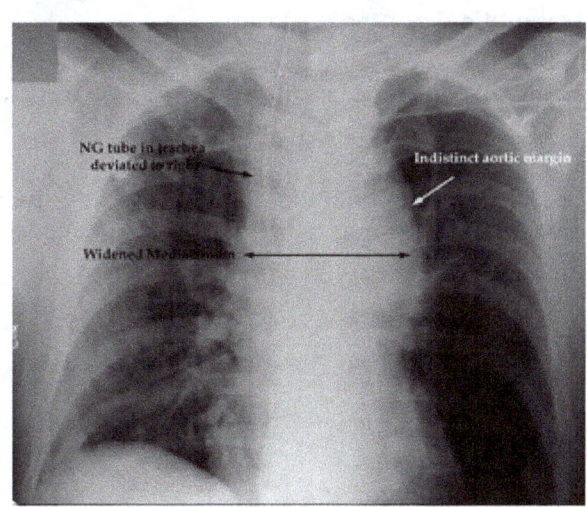

CXR demonstrating features of aortic injury

CT appearances:

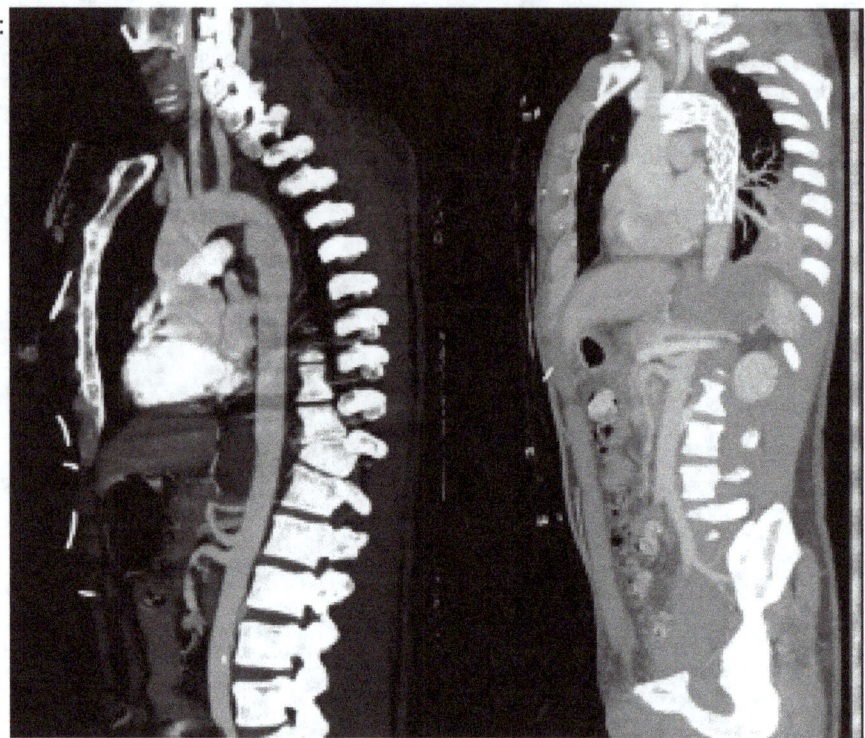

CT imaging of aortic disruption secondary to trauma (left) and subsequently following endovascular repair (right)

Management:
- Insert an A line in the right arm
- Strict blood pressure control
- Consider systemic analgesia
- Judicious fluid resuscitation, caution not to over transfuse
- Keep the patient as calm as possible to prevent stress and hypertension
- Urgent discussion with vascular surgeons and interventional radiology for definitive management (open surgical repair vs endovascular repair)

The majority of traumatic aortic injuries are managed by placement of an intra-aortic stent in the descending aorta (shown above). The stent is deployed via the femoral artery and often occludes the left subclavian artery, hence the need to monitor systemic blood pressure on the right arm when possible.

Traumatic diaphragm rupture

Most commonly, diaphragm rupture occurs secondary to blunt trauma involving high energy transfer or crush injuries. However, if you do have a patient with a penetrating injury to the flank or upper abdomen with evidence of blood above and below the diaphragm then a diaphragmatic injury should also be suspected. Furthermore, it is important in any penetrating torso injury to always consider the possibility of pathology within both the abdomen and the thoracic cavity. CT scans don't always demonstrate smaller defects and they may only be detected during video-assisted thoracoscopic surgery (VATS) exploration.

The only evidence of diaphragm rupture might be an ill-defined hemidiaphragm on a chest x-ray and this may only be evident later on. Right sided rupture is particularly hard to recognise due to the presence of the liver below and the absence of herniation of bowel into the thoracic cage. Any suspicion should therefore be discussed with thoracic surgeons. Even if they do not require intervention at the time, these patients are often followed up with repeat imaging to monitor for any progression of small defects.

The accompanying *eLearning Module 8* shows an example of a patient undergoing VATS repair of a ruptured diaphragm.

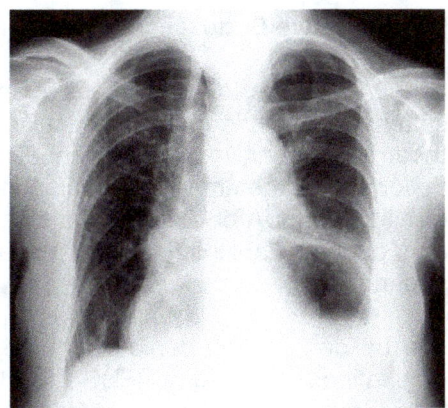

CXR of a patient with a ruptured diaphragm

Systemic air embolism

This is a relatively unknown sequela of severe thoracic injuries but is associated with a high mortality. It is associated with 4-14% of severe lung trauma, 67% of which is penetrating and the remainder contusions.

Most commonly, systemic air embolism occurs when patients have sustained injuries to the pulmonary veins and associated airways. These patients are often hypovolaemic with low pressure in their venous system. As air is introduced into the thoracic cavity, particularly if the patient is receiving positive-pressure ventilation, it can enter the circulation down a pressure gradient. This condition should be suspected if there are significant chest injuries, hypotension, blood in the airways or the ET tube or if there is a sudden collapse post intubation. Thought should be given to selectively ventilating the 'good' lung in these circumstances.

Diagnosis
- AIR in vessels – retinal, ABG
- Bubbles on transoesophageal echocardiogram
- Typically made during resuscitative thoracotomy

Management
- Give 100% oxygen
- Selective ventilation of 'good' lung
- Avoid high inflation pressures
- Emergent/resuscitative thoracotomy
    - Hilar clamping - prevents air entering the circulation
    - Lung repair

Resuscitative Endovascular Balloon Occlusion of the Aorta (REBOA)

REBOA involves the placement of an endovascular balloon inside the aorta to stem bleeding in patients suffering traumatic cardiac arrest or massive haemorrhage. This gives time for transfer to the operating theatre for definitive management. Its use is currently undergoing a multicentre trial within the UK, in which major trauma centres are participating. As discussed previously, the ERC guidelines recommend the use of either REBOA or direct aortic cross clamping as a last resort measure in patients with exsanguinating and uncontrollable infra-diaphragmatic torso haemorrhage.[1] Neither method has been shown to be superior.[3]

The balloon can be deployed in three zones within the aorta depending on where the haemorrhage is originating. When using REBOA for thoracic haemorrhage the balloon should be deployed in zone 1 (see figure below).[22] This extends from the origin of the left subclavian artery to the coeliac artery. There is currently limited evidence for its use in the hospital setting, however, the military are using it in the pre-hospital setting.

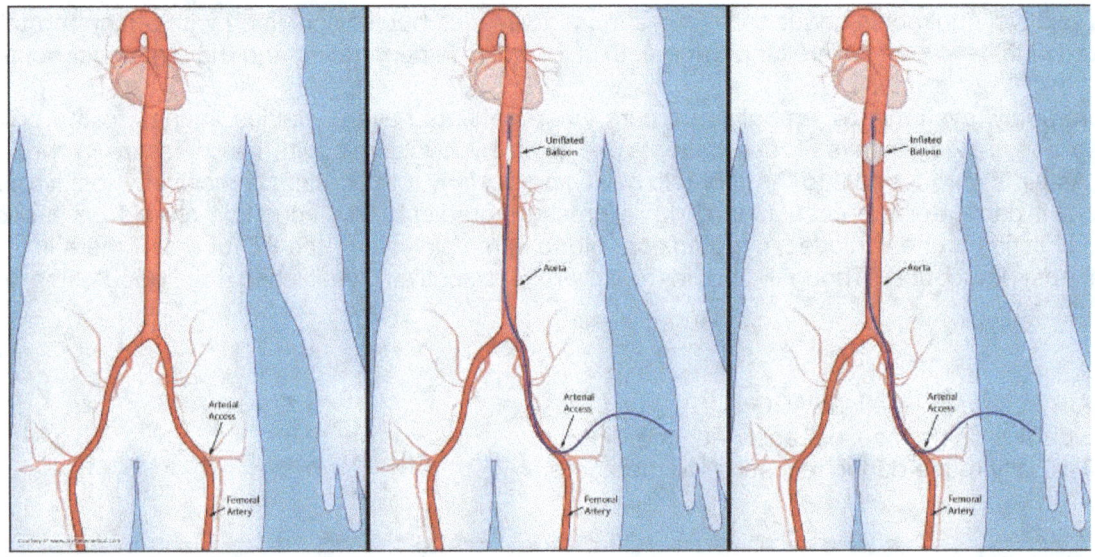

Schematic of zone 1 resuscitative endovascular balloon occlusion of the aorta, showing access and balloon deployment in the aorta (courtesy of Prytime Medical)
(Paul Rees et al. J R Army Med Corps 2018;164:72-76)[22]

Summary

We hope this chapter has made you more aware of some of the rare but catastrophic complications of chest trauma. Although definitive management often requires specialist teams, by suspecting these injuries when faced with the relevant patterns of injury, you can hopefully pre-empt such issues and obtain appropriate investigations. With the ability to perform CT scans easily, it is a key tool in helping to delineate injuries and direct further management so diagnoses won't be missed, and relevant teams can be involved early.

MOULAGES: PUTTING IT ALL INTO PRACTICE

eLearning Module 9

The best way for you to prepare for managing these patients is to practice moulages with the wider team present. In this way, you will become familiar with your equipment, the resuscitative thoracotomy protocols and your individual roles. Everyone will also appreciate how one another fits into the process and, particularly in these scenarios, how the cardiothoracic or general surgeons integrate into your trauma team. This method of learning and developing your respective teams is vital given the low volume yet high stake nature of these injuries. It goes without saying that real life patients should not be the testing ground for new skills, techniques or protocols. As far as possible, these should be practised in simulation with immediate feedback and subsequent refinement.

eLearning Module 9 has some video examples of moulages that we have run. During the interactive part of the course we aim to spend a reasonable amount of time taking you through different scenarios, but it is key that you then go back to your respective teams and build these into your own departmental training.

In particular, you should practise the following scenarios:

1. Standby call for arrested patient with penetrating trauma
2. Standby call for arrested patient who has had a pre-hospital resuscitative thoracotomy
3. Penetrating trauma patient who arrests in the emergency department
4. Standby call for a hypotensive penetrating trauma patient

A debrief and feedback session is as important as the scenario itself and we would encourage practice in large enough groups that a couple of people can observe each simulation and feedback to the group. Feedback should focus on the topics in the 'top tips' box below.

Top tips
Key elements of a successful RT moulage:
- ☑ Pre-allocation of roles
- ☑ Operators scrubbed and prepared (if relevant)
- ☑ Clear team leader with active followership
- ☑ Timely decision making
- ☑ Resuscitative thoracotomy protocol instigated once arrest confirmed
- ☑ **TRAUMATIC CROSS** time out at 10 minutes
- ☑ Effective resource coordination including facilitating onward transfer

HUMAN FACTORS IN RESUSCITATIVE THORACOTOMY

eLearning Module 10

Throughout your training you will have attended many courses that have practical or simulated elements. It always looks so easy in the simulation suite, but then when you are faced with the same situation in real life it doesn't work quite how you'd practised. So why does this happen? The answer is human factors. In healthcare, human factors are the non-technical factors which impact patient care and contribute to up to 70% of incidents.

To diminish the impact of human factors on patient outcomes, we need to work out how we are going to work better together and recreate what we've practised in training. An important step is to acknowledge that things do go wrong. No one comes to work intending to make mistakes or cause harm, however, as individuals or as a team, we are not always going to be perfect. *eLearning module 11* discusses how the airline industry is at the forefront of recognising these facts. Furthermore, people need to feel that they can report errors or near misses so that we can all learn from them or find ways to mitigate them. This is something we are less good at in healthcare. By acknowledging that mistakes can happen, we can put in barriers or mechanisms to prevent them. For example, we can use protocols or checklists to ensure that nothing is overlooked in stressful situations. Team work is also crucial during such times.

eLearning module 11 includes a widely viewed video on the tragic course of events that lead to the death of Elaine Bromiley. The case highlights some key human factors that often negatively impact patient care. There was a loss of situational awareness, no clear leadership, actions were not in line with established emergency protocols and a culture in which nurses were not listened to when they tried to speak up. There are key lessons to be learnt from this unfortunate case.

What do we have to do in emergency situations to make sure that we get the best outcomes?

There needs to be a good team leader, as many people as possible need to be conscious of the bigger picture and, as clinicians, we need to consider all possible diagnoses. Emergency protocols should be in place for both common and high-acuity low-occurrence (HALO) situations that are well versed and regularly practised. Hierarchies should be flattened so that anyone can feel empowered to speak up and let the team leader know their thoughts and concerns.

When the culture is not quite right, it can be hard for team members to feel they can speak up, particularly if it is to suggest that perhaps something has been missed or not considered. This may be a result of the systems that we work in or particular individuals leading a team. Whilst the hope is that there will be a cultural change in medicine to breakdown these barriers, it is also worth considering what any team member can do to raise their concerns.

There is a four-step process that can be utilised to approach these conversations or challenge authority without causing conflict; repeat, question, suggest and challenge. In a stepwise fashion one moves through the four stages until the concern has been acknowledged and taken into account. The first two stages give prompts and opportunities for the team leader to think through the situation and hopefully come to your conclusions for themselves. The third offers your ideas in a non-confrontational way and, finally, if you feel they still haven't taken on board your concerns, the fourth stage is the only point where you are actually challenging their authority. This last stage may be the only way to ensure the patient's safety and a positive outcome.

For example, if during a traumatic arrest with penetrating chest injuries the team is continuing to proceed as if it were a medical arrest with external chest compressions only, the following could be verbalised to the team leader:

1. Repeat "you think that we should just keep massaging"
2. Question "are you sure we should just keep massaging"
3. Suggest "well we could try a resuscitative thoracotomy"
4. Challenge "I really think we should do a thoracotomy"

Common pitfalls in resuscitation situations:

The table below has some common pitfalls in these scenarios with suggested solutions.

	Issues	Solutions
Environment	Non-uniform/complex environment	*Standardisation **and/or** thorough induction*
	High staff turnover and assumption of knowledge	*Discuss equipment and protocols with all new staff*
	Fatigue, noise, stress	*Supportive working environment and breaks* *Minimal distractions, no unnecessary team members/conversations*
Communication and Teamwork	Multiple, unfamiliar teams attending the ED	*Acknowledge and orientate them* *Organise simulation training together* *Use of communication boards*
	Poor communication, hierarchy and a culture not conducive to speaking up or learning from errors	*Strive for culture change* *Encourage participation from the whole team "does anyone have anything they would like to add"* *Team training* *Supportive group discussions/reflections on errors and learning points*
	Vague instructions or leadership "can someone get me the…"	*Name individuals for tasks* *Clear instruction/delegation*
	Lack of awareness of the wider picture	*Briefing to the whole team e.g. before an intervention* *10 minute time out*
	Team leader fixated on difficult tasks/procedures	*Hands-off team leader* *Acknowledge that operators doing difficult tasks should not be multitasking and trying to lead the team*

Leadership and active followership

A team approach is a key element of human factors training. Our protocol enables the team leader to remain hands-off and maintain a global overview of the resuscitation and it is important that they resist the temptation to intervene. If necessary, the leader can assign another individual to help a struggling team member. The leader needs to make clear decisions, assign tasks and remain calm. It is clearly important that they have a good technical knowledge and, given the high-acuity low-occurrence of these resuscitations, this should be a senior doctor with relevant experience. As we have discussed, they need to be authoritative but open to suggestions from the whole team.

Active followership is vital to ensure that communication is maintained with the team leader. Team members should carry out their assigned tasks but report back to the team leader, for example to inform them that the ET tube is in and you have bilateral air entry and end-tidal CO2. They should support the team leader and defer any decision making to them unless clinically inappropriate. Finally, it is important that all suggestions are made to the team leader to prevent multiple separate discussions developing within the team. Active followership in itself is a skill and simulation training allows all members to adopt and cultivate this practice.

Avoiding fixation errors

Fixation errors negatively impact many stressful situations and should be avoided. They may take several forms:
- **'This and only this'**
    - Persistent failure to revise diagnosis/plan, despite contrary evidence
    - Available evidence interpreted to fit
    - Attention allocated to minor aspect of problem
- **'Anything but this'**
    - Persistent failure to commit to definitive treatment
    - Extended search for information, without addressing problem
- **'Everything is ok'**
    - Persistent belief that there is no problem, despite evidence that there is
    - Abnormalities attributed to artefact/transients
    - Failure to declare emergency or request/accept help

Obviously, in the context of traumatic arrest secondary to penetrating chest trauma, any of the above could result in a poor outcome if a resuscitative thoracotomy is delayed or not performed.

Fixation errors can be prevented with thorough training, teamwork, good leadership that encourages contribution from the whole team and use of cognitive aids (discussed below). Importantly, by training as a team, all members should develop an understanding of the protocol, each role and the equipment. This awareness helps individuals to support each other, pick up on any concerns or issues that another team member may be experiencing and avoid fixation errors.

Use of cognitive aids

Emergencies are not the time to test your memory. When faced with an uncommon scenario, mistakes are far more likely to be made if the team is trying to recall a training session from months back, rather than following a printed pathway. For the majority of hospitals in the world, resuscitative thoracotomies are a prime example. Guidelines and visual aids provide structure and a user-friendly way to ensure that all key aspects are considered, important safety steps are taken and nothing is forgotten. This course centres around a clear protocol supported by posters, a flipchart and checklists, including the 10 minute time out. These aids need to always be accessible in a suitable location, for example a flipchart on top of the resuscitative thoracotomy set.

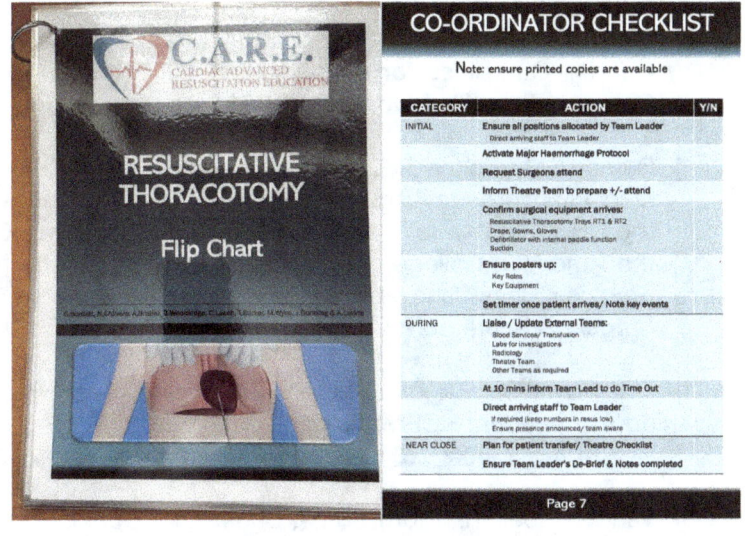

Conclusions

Human factors play a huge role in these high-acuity low-occurrence scenarios. Teams should strive to develop a supportive and reflective culture, like that of the airline industry, to facilitate the best possible care for these patients. Many of the issues discussed can be mitigated to a large extent by good training involving all team members. Unfortunately, there is very little standardisation between centres and this is compounded by high staff turnover and frequent rotation of training doctors between hospitals. This is where the practical elements of this course can really help to develop your individual teams and should be consolidated by ongoing training in your own centres.

REFERENCES

[1] Lott C, Truhlář A, Alfonzo A, Barelli A, González-Salvado V, Hinkelbein J, et al. European Resuscitation Council Guidelines 2021: Cardiac arrest in special circumstances, *Resuscitation*. 2021; article in press.

[2] Truhlář A, Deakin CD, Soar J, Khalifa GE, Alfonzo A, Bierens JJ, et al. European Resuscitation Council Guidelines for Resuscitation 2015: Section 4. Cardiac arrest in special circumstances. *Resuscitation*. 2015 Oct;95:148-201.

[3] Bulger EM, Perina DG, Qasim Z, Beldowicz B, Brenner M, Guyette F, et al. Clinical use of resuscitative endovascular balloon occlusion of the aorta (REBOA) in civilian trauma systems in the USA, 2019: a joint statement from the American College of Surgeons Committee on Trauma, the American College of Emergency Physicians, the National Association of Emergency Medical Services Physicians and the National Association of Emergency Medical Technicians. *Trauma Surgery & Acute Care Open*. 2019;4:e000376.

[4] The Royal College of Emergency Medicine. Best Practice Guideline - Traumatic cardiac arrest in adults. London: RCEM; 2019. Available from: https://www.rcem.ac.uk/docs/RCEM%20Guidance/RCEM_Traumatic%20cardiac%20arrest_Sept%202019%20FINAL.pdf

[5] Vanden Hoek TL, Morrison LJ, Shuster M, Donnino M, Sinz E, Lavonas EJ, et al. Part 12: Cardiac Arrest in Special Situations: 2010 American Heart Association Guidelines for Cardiopulmonary Resuscitation and Emergency Cardiovascular Care. *Circulation*. 2010 Nov 2;122(18 Suppl 3):S829-61.

[6] Lavonas EJ, Drennan IR, Gabrielli A, Heffner AC, Hoyte CO, Orkin AM, et al. Part 10: Special Circumstances of Resuscitation: 2015 American Heart Association Guidelines Update for Cardiopulmonary Resuscitation and Emergency Cardiovascular Care. *Circulation*. 2015 Nov 3;132(18 Suppl 2):S501-18.

[7] Hopson LR, Hirsh E, Delgado J, Domeier RM, McSwain NE Jr, Krohmer J, et al. Guidelines for withholding or termination of resuscitation in prehospital traumatic cardiopulmonary arrest: a joint position paper from the National Association of EMS Physicians Standards and Clinical Practice Committee and the American College of Surgeons Committee on Trauma. *Prehosp Emerg Care*. 2003 Jan-Mar;7(1):141-6.

[8] Working Group, Ad Hoc Subcommittee on Outcomes, American College of Surgeons - Committee on Trauma. Practice management guidelines for emergency department thoracotomy. *J Am Coll Surg*. 2001 Sep;193(3):303-9.

[9] Seamon MJ, Haut ER, Van Arendonk K, Barbosa RR, Chiu WC, Dente CJ, et al. An evidence-based approach to patient selection for emergency department thoracotomy: A practice management guideline from the Eastern Association for the Surgery of Trauma. *J Trauma Acute Care Surg*. 2015 Jul;79(1):159-73.

[10] The Royal Melbourne Hospital Emergency Department Advisory Committee on Trauma. Emergency Department Thoracotomy Guideline. Melbourne: The Royal Melbourne Hospital Trauma Service; 2018. Available from: https://www.thermh.org.au/sites/default/files/media/documents/clinical/Emergency%20Department%20Thoracotomy%20Guideline.pdf

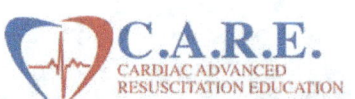

REFERENCES

[11] South Yorkshire Major Trauma Operational Delivery Network. Network Guidelines for Resuscitative Thoracotomy (Adults and Paediatrics). Sheffield: SYMT ODN; 2018. Available from: http://www.csodn.nhs.uk/wp-content/uploads/SYMT-ODN-Guideline-for-Resuscitative-Thoracotomy-V3.0.pdf

[12] Wise D, Davies G, Coats T, Lockey D, Hyde J, Good A. Emergency thoracotomy: "how to do it". *Emerg Med J*. 2005 Jan;22(1):22-4.

[13] Faculty of Pre-Hospital Care The Royal College of Surgeons Edinburgh. Consensus Statement 2018 Management of Traumatic Cardiac Arrest. Edinburgh: FPHC; 2018. Available from: https://fphc.rcsed.ac.uk/media/2577/tca-submission-oct-2018.pdf

[14] American College of Surgeons Committee on Trauma. Advanced Trauma Life Support Student Course Manual. 10th Edition. Chicago: American College of Surgeons; 2018.

[15] ETC CMC. European Trauma Course: The Team Approach. 4th Edition. Antwerp: ETCO; 2018.

[16] Feliciano DV. Cardiac, Great Vessel and Pulmonary Injuries. In: Rasmussen TE, Tai NR, editors. Rich's Vascular Trauma. 3rd Edition. Philadelphia: Elsevier; 2016. p. 73-99.

[17] Warrington SJ, Mahajan K. Cardiac Trauma. In: StatPearls [Internet]. Treasure Island: StatPearls Publishing; 2020. Available from: https://www.ncbi.nlm.nih.gov/books/NBK430725/

[18] Wilson A, Wall MJ Jr, Maxson R, Mattox K. The pulmonary hilum twist as a thoracic damage control procedure. *Am J Surg*. 2003 Jul;186(1):49-52.

[19] University Hospitals Coventry and Warwickshire NHS Trust. Major Trauma? Major Haemorrhage? Guideline. Coventry: UHCW; 2019.

[20] Frerk C, Mitchell VS, McNarry AF, Mendonca C, Bhagrath R, Patel A, et al. Difficult Airway Society 2015 guidelines for management of unanticipated difficult intubation in adults. *Br J Anaesth*. 2015 Dec;115(6):827–848.

[21] University Hospitals Coventry and Warwickshire NHS Trust. Multiple Rib Fracture Pain Management Algorithm. Coventry: UHCW; 2020.

[22] Rees P, Waller B, Buckley AM, Doran C, Bland S, Scott T, et al. REBOA at Role 2 Afloat: resuscitative endovascular balloon occlusion of the aorta as a bridge to damage control surgery in the military maritime setting. *J R Army Med Corps*. 2018 May;164(2):72-76.

NOTES

NOTES

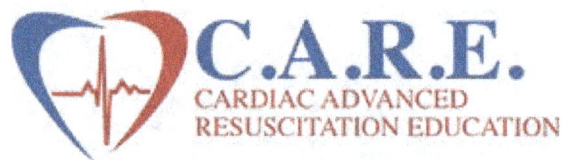

www.csu-als.org